Comorbidity of Addictive and Psychiatric Disorders

The Journal of Addictive Diseases series:*
(formerly Advances in Alcohol & Substance Abuse series)

- *Behavioral and Biochemical Issues in Substance Abuse**
- *Cocaine, AIDS, and Intravenous Drug Use**
- *What Works in Drug Abuse Epidemiology**
- *Cocaine: Physiological and Physiopathological Effects**
- *Recent Advances in the Biology of Alcoholism*
- *The Effects of Maternal Alcohol and Drug Abuse on the Newborn*
- *Evaluation of Drug Treatment Programs*
- *Current Controversies in Alcoholism*
- *Federal Priorities in Funding Alcohol and Drug Abuse Programs*
- *Psychosocial Constructs of Alcoholism and Substance Abuse*
- *The Addictive Behaviors*
- *Conceptual Issues in Alcoholism and Substance Abuse*
- *Dual Addiction: Pharmacological Issues in the Treatment of Concomitant Alcoholism and Drug Abuse*
- *Cultural and Sociological Aspects of Alcholism and Substance Abuse*
- *Alcohol and Drug Abuse in the Affluent*
- *Alcohol and Substance Abuse in Adolescence*
- *Controversies in Alcoholism and Substance Abuse*
- *Alcohol and Substance Abuse in Women and Children*
- *Cocaine: Pharmacology, Addiction, and Therapy*
- *Children of Alcoholics*
- *Pharmacological Issues in Alcohol and Substance Abuse*
- *AIDS and Substance Abuse*
- *Alcohol Research from Bench to Bedside*
- *Addiction Potential of Abused Drugs and Drug Classes*
- *Comorbidity of Addictive and Psychiatric Disorders*

Comorbidity of Addictive and Psychiatric Disorders

Norman S. Miller, MD
Guest Editor

Barry Stimmel, MD
Editor

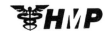

The Haworth Medical Press
an Imprint of
The Haworth Press, Inc.
New York • London • Norwood (Australia)

Published by

The Haworth Medical Press, 10 Alice Street, Binghamton, NY 13904-1580.

The Haworth Medical Press is an imprint of The Haworth Press, Inc., 10 Alice Street, Binghamton, NY 13904-1580 USA.

Comorbidity of Addictive and Psychiatric Disorders has also been published as *Journal of Addictive Diseases,* Volume 12, Number 3, 1993.

Library of Congress Cataloging–in–Publication Data

Comorbidity of addictive and psychiatric disorders / Norman S. Miller, guest editor ; Barry Stimmel, editor.
    p. cm.
    "Has also been published as Journal of addictive diseases, volume 12, number 3, 1993"–T.p. verso.
    Includes bibliographical references.
    ISBN 1-56024-457-7 (alk. paper)
    1. Dual diagnosis. I. Miller, Norman S. II. Stimmel, Barry, 1939- .
    [DNLM: 1. Behavior, Addictive–epidemiology, 2. Mental Disorders–epidemiology. 3. Comorbidity. W1 JO533PU v. 12, no.3 1993 / WM 176 C735 1993]
RC564.68.C65 1993
616.86–dc20
DNLM/DLC
for Library of Congress   93-24682
                                                                     CIP

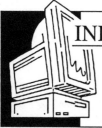

INDEXING & ABSTRACTING

Contributions to this publication are selectively indexed or abstracted in print, electronic, online, or CD-ROM version(s) of the reference tools and information services listed below. This list is current as of the copyright date of this publication. See the end of this section for additional notes.

- *Abstracts in Anthropology,* Baywood Publishing Company, 26 Austin Avenue, P.O. Box 337, Amityville, NY 11701

- *Abstracts of Research in Pastoral Care & Counseling,* Loyola College, 7135 Minstrel Way, Suite 101, Columbia, MD 21045

- *Alcohol Clinical Update "Abstracts Section,"* Project Cork Institute, 14 S. Main Street, Suite 2F, Hanover, NH 03755-2015

- *ALCONARC Database,* Swedish Council for Information on Alcohol and Other Drugs, Box 27302, S-102 54 Stockholm, Sweden

- *Biosciences Information Service of Biological Abstracts (BIOSIS),* Biosciences Information Service, 2100 Arch Street, Philadelphia, PA 19103-1399

- *Bulletin Signaletique,* INIST/CNRS-Service Gestion des Documents Primaires, 2 allee du Parc de Brabois, F-54514 Vandoeuvre-les-Nancy, Cedex, France

- *Cambridge Scientific Abstracts, Health & Safety Science Abstracts,* Cambridge Information Group, 7200 Wisconsin Avenue #601, Bethesda, MD 20814

- *Child Development Abstracts & Bibliography,* University of Kansas, 2 Bailey Hall, Lawrence, KS 66045

- *Criminal Justice Abstracts,* Willow Tree Press, 15 Washington Street, 4th Floor, Newark, NJ 07102

- *Criminal Justice Periodical Index,* University Microfilms, Inc., 300 North Zeeb Road, Ann Arbor, MI 48106

- *Criminology, Penology and Police Science Abstracts,* Kugler Publication bv, P.O. Box 516, 1180 AM-Amstelveen, The Netherlands

- *Current Awareness in Biological Sciences (C.A.B.S),* 132 New Walk, Leicester LE1 7QQ, UK

(continued)

- *Excerpta Medica/Electronic Publishing Division,* Elsevier Science Publishers, 655 Avenue of the Americans, New York, NY 10010

- *Index Medicus/MEDLINE,* National Library of Medicine, 8600 Rockville Pike, Bethesda, MD 20894

- *Index to Periodical Articles Related to Law,* University of Texas, 727 East 26th Street, Austin, TX 78705

- *International Pharmaceutical Abstracts,* American Society of Hospital Pharmacists, 7272 Wisconsin Avenue, Bethesda, MD 20814

- *Inventory of Marriage and Family Literature (online and hard copy),* National Council on Family Relations, 3989 Central Avenue NE, Suite 550, Minneapolis, MN 55421

- *Mental Health Abstracts (online through DIALOG),* IFI/Plenum Data Company, 3202 Kirkwood Highway, Wilmington, DE 19808

- *Medication Use Studies (MUST) Database,* School of Pharmacy, The University of Mississippi, University, MS 38677

- *NIAAA Alcohol and Alcohol Problems Science Database (ETOH),* National Institute on Alcohol Abuse and Alcoholism, 1400 Eye Street NW, Suite 600, Washington, DC 20090-1600

- *Psychological Abstracts (PsycINFO),* American Psychological Association, P.O. Box 91600, Washington, DC 20090-1600

- *SilverPlatter Information Inc.,* Imformation Resources Group, 101 West Walnut Street, Suite 200, Pasadena, CA 91103

- *Social Planning/Policy & Development Abstracts (SOPODA),* Sociological Abstracts, Inc., P.O. Box 22206, San Diego, CA 92122-0206

- *Social Work Research & Abstracts,* National Association of Social Workers, 750 First Street NW, 8th Floor, Washington, DC 20002

- *Sociological Abstracts (SA),* Sociological Abstracts, Inc., P.O. Box 22206, San Diego, CA 92122-0206

- *SOMED (social medicine) Database,* Institute fur Dokumentation, Postfach 20 10 12, D-4800 Bielefeld 1, Germany

- *Studies on Women Abstracts,* Carfax Publishing Company, P.O. Box 25, Abingdon, Oxfordshire, OX14 3UE, England

(continued)

SPECIAL BIBLIOGRAPHIC NOTES

related to indexing and abstracting

❏ indexing/abstracting services in this list will also cover material in the "separate" that is co-published simultaneously with Haworth's special thematic journal issue or DocuSerial. Indexing/abstracting usually covers material at the article/chapter level.

❏ monographic co-editions are intended for either non-subscribers or libraries which intend to purchase a second copy for their circulating collections.

❏ monographic co-editions are reported to all jobbers/wholesalers/approval plans. The source journal is listed as the "series" to assist the prevention of duplicate purchasing in the same manner utilized for books-in-series.

❏ to facilitate user/access services all indexing/abstracting services are encouraged to utilize the co-indexing entry note indicated at the bottom of the first page of each article/chapter/contribution.

❏ this is intended to assist a library user of any reference tool (whether print, electronic, online, or CD-ROM) to locate the monographic version if the library has purchased this version but not a subscription to the source journal.

❏ individual articles/chapters in any Haworth publication are also available through the Haworth Document Delivery Services (HDDS).

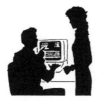

Comorbidity of Addictive and Psychiatric Disorders

CONTENTS

EDITORIAL: A Tale of Two Diagnoses: Revisited   1
Norman S. Miller

Comorbidity of Psychiatric and Alcohol/Drug Disorders:
    Interactions and Independent Status   5
Norman S. Miller

Genetic and Family Studies in Psychiatric Illness
    and Alcohol and Drug Dependence   17
Stephen H. Dinwiddie
Theodore Reich

Hypothesized Neurochemical Models for Psychiatric
    Syndromes in Alcohol and Drug Dependence   29
Irl L. Extein
Mark S. Gold

The Epidemiology of the Comorbidity of Psychiatric
    and Addictive Disorders: A Critical Review   45
Valerie D. Raskin
Norman S. Miller

Evaluation and Acute Management of Psychotic
    Symptomatology in Alcohol and Drug Addictions   59
James Fine
Norman S. Miller

Affective and Anxiety Disorders and Alcohol and Drug
    Dependence: Diagnosis and Treatment   73
Robert M. Anthenelli
Marc A. Schuckit

Pathological Gambling, Eating Disorders,
    and the Psychoactive Substance Use Disorders   89
        Henry R. Lesieur
        Sheila B. Blume

The Dually Diagnosed Patient with Psychotic Symptoms   103
        Richard K. Ries

Outpatient vs. Inpatient Treatment for the Chronically
    Mentally Ill with Substance Use Disorders   123
        Lial Kofoed

An Integrated Psychology for the Addictions:
    Beyond the Self-Medication Hypothesis   139
        R. Jeffrey Goldsmith

Pharmacotherapy of Psychiatric Syndromes with Comorbid
    Chemical Dependence   155
        David R. Gastfriend

SELECTIVE GUIDE TO CURRENT REFERENCE
SOURCES ON TOPICS DISCUSSED IN THIS ISSUE
    Comorbidity of Addictive and Psychiatric Disorders   171
        Lynn Kasner Morgan
        James E. Raper, Jr

Comorbidity of Addictive and Psychiatric Disorders

ABOUT THE GUEST EDITOR

Norman S. Miller, MD, is Associate Professor of Psychiatry, Chief of Addiction Programs, and Associate Professor of Neurology at the University of Illinois at Chicago College of Medicine. He has extensive teaching, administrative, and professional experience and has published many journal articles and book chapters. An editorial board member or reviewer for a number of professional journals, Dr. Miller is a Fellow in the American Psychopathological Association and a member of the American Psychiatric Association, the American Society for Addiction Medicine, and the American Academy of Psychiatrists in Alcoholism and Addictions and serves on several national professional committees. He is also Chief of the Section for the Dual Diagnosis Program for the West Side Veterans Administration Medical Center.

Comorbidity
of Addictive
and Psychiatric
Disorders

EDITORIAL

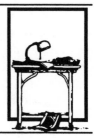

A Tale of Two Diagnoses: Revisited

The field of addiction has come full circle. It now appears that the "psychiatric" explanation for addictive disorders has returned.

Norman S. Miller is affiliated with the Department of Psychiatry, University of Illinois at Chicago, West Side VA Medical Center, Chicago, IL.

Requests for reprints should be addressed to Norman S. Miller, MD, Department of Psychiatry, University of Illinois at Chicago, 912 South Wood Street, Chicago, IL 60612.

[Haworth co-indexing entry note]: "Editorial: A Tale of Two Diagnoses: Revisited." Miller, Norman S. Co-published simultaneously in *Journal of Addictive Diseases,* (The Haworth Press, Inc.) Vol. 12, No. 3, 1993, pp. 1-4; and: *Comorbidity of Addictive and Psychiatric Disorders* (Ed: Norman S. Miller, and Barry Stimmel) The Haworth Press, Inc., 1993, pp. 1-4. Multiple copies of this article/chapter may be purchased from The Haworth Document Delivery Center. Call 1-800-3-HAWORTH (1-800-342-9678) between 9:00 - 5:00(EST) and ask for DOCUMENT DELIVERY CENTER.

1

For years, traditional psychiatric methods have been employed by psychiatrists in the diagnosis and treatment of addictive disorders with limited success, and considerable untoward results. The practice of assigning an underlying cause to abnormal drinking and drug use by the psychiatrist conforms to the user's dynamics to rationalize and avoid facing the central problem of addiction. The major consequence is that the addict is distracted from proper diagnosis and treatment, and often becomes worse. In the end, neither the psychiatrist nor the patient is satisfied, and is at odds with mistrust and blame towards each other.[1,2]

The addiction field has grown up essentially aside from the psychiatric profession with some notable exceptions, namely, Drs. William Silkworth, Harry Tiebolt and Ruth Fox among others along the way. The movement of Alcoholics Anonymous has provided an accurate depiction of the addictive behaviors and psychic of the alcoholic (and drug addict). AA importantly employs the "medical model" of addiction for the purpose of treatment of alcoholism (drug addiction). Drug addiction is emphasized not only because the majority of contemporary alcoholics are addicted to other drugs but also the co-founders of AA were addicted to various drugs during their alcoholic years. Currently, millions of alcoholics and drug addicts are recovering in AA throughout the world. Other similar organizations using the principles of AA have arisen such as Narcotics Anonymous, and are having success as well.[3]

Until recently, psychiatry appeared content with avoiding the addictive disorders. Psychiatry is now experiencing a reentry into the diagnosis and treatment of addictive disorders. The reasons are complex but are attributable to the inclusion of independent and exclusionary criteria for substance use disorders in DSM-III and DSM-III-R, explosion of alcohol and drug disorders in psychiatric populations and the shrinking pie of reimbursement that has kindled competition between psychiatry and the addiction treatment establishment.[1]

The addiction treatment establishment evolved largely because of the AA movement, the unwillingness of psychiatry to diagnosis and treat addictive disorders and the more tolerant and accepting attitudes by employers, courts and health professionals (physicians largely notwithstanding). The minority of the physicians who have supported the treatment of addictive disorders formed the professional organization that is now called the American Society of Addiction Medicine.[4]

As psychiatry moves into the addiction field, i.e., added qualification for addiction psychiatry to the American Board of Psychiatry and Neurology, it continues to emphasize traditional psychiatric methods. The focus is on the diagnosis of "psychiatric disorders" in alcoholics and drug addicts as always and how psychiatric treatments affect the outcome of the addict. What is missing is the adoption of the skills and techniques of addiction treatment that have been developed over the past 50 years. Psychiatry has not changed its views and approach to addictive disorders but merely has revisited an old problem.

The tensions remain, and most unfortunately, for the alcoholic and drug addict. It is this editor's opinion that the resistance to having psychiatrists learn and use addiction methods in the treatment of addictive disorders is minimal. On the other hand, the resistance of the psychiatrists to incorporating addiction treatment methods into their practice is enormous. Curiously, the addiction treatment establishment has never had much objection to diagnosing independent psychiatric disorders in addicted patients, and still does not.

Studies have clearly established that alcohol and drug addiction can generate psychiatric symptoms that resolve with abstinence and specific treatment of the addiction, thereby establishing addiction as an independent disorder. No studies have shown that psychiatric symptoms or underlying disorders cause addiction to alcohol and drugs. Although studies are lacking, clinical experience strongly suggests that concomitant treatment of independent psychiatric disorders will improve the prognosis of the addictive disorder. Studies have shown that the prognosis for treatment of independent psychiatric disorders remains poor without specific treatment of the independent addictive disorders. What we have learned over the past 50 years is that treatment of the addictive disorders as independent diseases carries the best prognosis whether or not another psychiatric disorder is present.[4,5]

Norman S. Miller, MD

SELECTED BIBLIOGRAPHY

1. Miller NS, Mahler JC, Belkin BM, Gold MS. Psychiatric diagnosis in alcohol and drug dependence. Annals of Clinical Psychiatry 1990; 3(1): 79-89.

2. Ries RK, Samson H. Substance abuse among inpatient psychiatric patients. Substance Abuse 1987; 8:28-34.

3. Alcoholics Anonymous Membership 1989 Survey. Alcoholics Anonymous World Services, Inc. Box 459, Grand Central Station, New York, NY 10163.

4. Harrison A, Hoffman NG, Sneed SG. Treatment Outcome. In Miller NS, (ed). 1991 Comprehensive Handbook of Drug and Alcohol Addiction. Marcel-Dekker, Inc. New York.

5. Blankfield A. Psychiatric symptoms in alcohol dependence. Diagnosis and treatment implications. Journal of Substance Abuse Treatment 1986; 3:275-278.

Comorbidity of Psychiatric and Alcohol/Drug Disorders: Interactions and Independent Status

Norman S. Miller, MD

SUMMARY. Dual diagnosis as interpreted in clinical psychiatric practice is often not what the term means-two independent disorders. Commonly, addiction disorders are attributed to self medicating of "underlying" psychiatric disorders, there by, a contingency status. However, studies and clinical addiction practice show that drug and alcohol addiction must be afforded an independent status before accurate assessment and assignment of interactions in dual diagnosis can be made in clinical conditions. Studies also show rates for psychiatric comorbidity are low in addiction populations and rates for addictive disorders are high in psychiatric populations. If the common denominator is taken as addiction, then the perspective of the setting and examiner become crucial in determining prevalence rates for both disorders. Most importantly, effective treatment of either disorder will not occur unless an agreement on an independent status is accepted for both addictive and psychiatric disorders in any patient population setting.

Norman S. Miller is affiliated with the Department of Psychiatry, University of Illinois at Chicago, West Side VA Medical Center, Chicago, IL.

Reprint requests should be addressed to Norman S. Miller, MD, Department of Psychiatry (M/C 913), University of Illinois at Chicago, 912 South Wood Street, Chicago, IL 60612.

[Haworth co-indexing entry note]: "Comorbidity of Psychiatric and Alcohol/ Drug Disorders: Interactions and Independent Status." Miller, Norman S. Co-published simultaneously in *Journal of Addictive Diseases,* (The Haworth Press, Inc.) Vol. 12, No. 3, 1993, pp. 5-16; and: *Comorbidity of Addictive and Psychiatric Disorders* (Ed: Norman S. Miller, and Barry Stimmel) The Haworth Press, Inc., 1993, pp. 5-16. Multiple copies of this article/chapter may be purchased from The Haworth Document Delivery Center. Call 1-800-3-HAWORTH (1-800-342-9678) between 9:00 - 5:00(EST) and ask for DOCUMENT DELIVERY CENTER.

STATEMENT OF THE ESSENTIALS

Definition of Dual Diagnosis

Definition and operationalization of diagnostic categories for alcohol and drug disorders are continuous sources of confusion for psychiatry and medicine. The origins of confusion are multifactorial, within and outside the purview of psychiatry and medicine, and attributable to attitudinal, philosophical, and empirical differences toward diagnosis and treatment of these disorders. In addition, the countertransference of stigma that all professionals project on the subject of "dual diagnosis" bears heavily on interpretation of clinical states. Of no small importance are the traditional tenets of disciplines that bar methodologies not germane to their diagnostic and treatment framework.[1]

A subset of "dual diagnosis" is examined pertaining to presence of alcohol and drug use and addiction in conjunction with a psychiatric disorder. Already, there is hesitancy in proceeding further without defining possible interactions between addiction and psychiatric disorders. Also, while not in subject of the review, the presence of an addictive disorder and a medical condition (prevalence rates in medical populations for alcoholics/drug addicts are 25-50%) would meet accepted requirements of a "dual diagnosis."

Terminology

Terms that have arisen as attempts at precise description of dual diagnosis are co-occurrence, coexistence, comorbidity, concurrent and simultaneous. Besides being hard to spell, they denote only that two or more conditions occur together without specifying when, why or how. The terms coexistence and comorbidity suffer from similar limitations in being difficult to operationalize; however, designating a condition as co-morbid does indicate that diseases or pathological states arise together. "Concurrent" is the occurrence of two conditions that co-vary over time but not at the same time, i.e., marijuana use precedes cocaine use, whereas "simultaneous" is the occurrence at the same time, such that alcohol and cocaine are used in the same individual overlapping in time. Importantly, all the terms do not specify the possible interactions between the conditions that occur in relation to each other.

Interactions in Dual Diagnosis

Perhaps the most poorly understood but an essential feature of dual diagnosis is the nature and direction of interactions between two or more conditions. While various schemes to define interactions have been proposed, no one approach is satisfactory in describing the dynamics of dually occurring conditions with alcohol/drug disorders. The terms "primary" and "secondary" are perhaps most commonly used, followed by "major" and "minor."[2]

Primary and secondary have multiple variations to their meanings that are often dependent on the perceptions of the user. Primary may mean "to cause" as in determining, or "to be central" as overriding to a secondary condition that is a direct result or indirect consequence. A simple example is alcohol inducing depression in single or repetitive doses where alcohol is the "cause of depression." Another more complex example is antisocial personality disorder as a risk factor for or "central" to alcohol and drug dependence as an overriding condition in the onset of alcohol use and dependence.

Another use of these terms are the temporal or chronological priority such as one condition occurring before the other in time. While one condition may precede another, there is no direct or obligatory causal relationship. However, it is often implied that the first condition will determine the overall course of the two illnesses. An example is a patient who develops a schizophrenic illness in adolescence, and later develops alcohol dependence as an adult. While both illnesses are chronic and progressive, the schizophrenic illness will "determine" the eventual clinical course even if the alcoholism is treated. An example of a "casual" relationship is anxiety arising in an alcoholic where alcoholism precedes and induces anxiety. Ultimately, the progression of the alcoholism will determine the prognosis of both disorders whether or not the anxiety is treated by other means.

Major and minor are less clearly defined terms and probably have more subjective than objective application in clinical and research settings. Major often implies a "big" or "troublesome" role in the clinical course that must be "dealt with" or treated before other conditions can be adequately treated. An example is a manic who is also alcoholic where the alcoholism must be treated in order to enhance compliance with chronic medications for mania. In this case the alcoholism is a major feature in the course of diagnosis and treatment of mania. An example of minor may be an anxiety disorder such as a phobia in alcoholic patients. The alcoholism is the crucial factor in the patient's clinical state but may intensify the phobia. While it may interfere with specific function, the phobia in the alcoholic is a minor condition that is not responsible for the preponderance of morbidity and potential mortality from the alcoholism.

The principle drawbacks to strict adherence to primary/secondary and major/minor determinations are that they work for some disorders and not for others and not all the time for any disorder. Furthermore, misapplications of these schemes arise because history will not always reveal which disorder has been currently predominating the clinical picture. Additionally, which disorder is predominating the clinical picture when two are actually present is not always ascertainable on cross sectional analysis. For instance, major depression generally has an exacerbating and remitting course, such that it may appear before an addictive disorder and not necessarily with it. If depression is present with alcoholism later in the course, the depression cannot be automatically assumed to be from a recurrent major depressive disorder, and it is statistically more likely to be due to alcohol consumption and addiction.

For major depression to be predominant in this case, one must assume there was a long, protracted course of depression or a timely recurrence of depression in the setting of active drinking. Commonly, in psychiatric practice recurrent major depression will be diagnosed in lieu of alcohol induced depression if one simply disregards alcoholism as a primary condition and etiologic to depression or simply if one does not know how to diagnosis alcoholism. The opposite error in diagnosis may occur in the alcoholic who is severely depressed in the setting of active drinking. Because major depression is common in the population, particularly in females, it must be considered that alcohol consumption/addiction is not totally causative of the depression, and that an independent major depression may be operative in the clinical picture.

Etiology of Psychiatric Symptoms

The erroneous assumption often leading to an incorrect diagnosis of major depression in the setting of active alcoholism is that depression causes or predisposes one to alcohol consumption.[3] Studies that examine in a controlled fashion the relationship between drinking and depression do not support this popular notion, and in fact demonstrate that alcoholics become more depressed when drinking and appear to drink despite alcohol-induced depression.[4] Moreover, it has been documented that alcohol consumption is negatively correlated with depression in nonalcoholics. While normals and nonalcoholic depressives receive enhanced mood and affect from drinking, their alcohol consumption actually decreases over time during depressive episodes. Similar results have been found for anxiety where nonalcoholic anxious people drink less, and alcoholics become more anxious the longer and more they drink. Moreover, both depressed and anxious alcoholics become less affected by these symptoms in proportion to their abstinence from alcohol.[4,5]

One understandable source for these commonly held beliefs is that alcoholics report drinking because of anxiety and depression.[3] However, controlled studies demonstrate that although alcoholics will report the need to drink when anxious and depressed, they become depressed and anxious to the point of suicide *after* and not preceding regular consumption of alcohol.[6] Paradoxically, after detoxification and abstinence, recall for the depressed and anxious moods in the setting of active drinking is poor but patients continue to attribute a therapeutic benefit on mood to the alcohol until the addict understands his or her addictive use of alcohol and drugs through treatment or self-help improvement.[6]

Moreover, there are other mental and neurological illnesses wherein the self-report is inconsistent with reality, i.e., hallucinations, delusions, confabulation in schizophrenia and Alzheimer's disease. Although we accept the self-report of these patients as their experience, we do not take what they report as consistent with reality. Similarly, the peculiar mental state of the alcoholic, while real to the drinker, does not conform to the observed clinical reality and experimental testing and should not be accepted at face value, as it often is without attendant risk of error.[6]

The commonly associated psychological states of denial, rationalization and minimization serve to distort perceptions and alter judgements of the alcoholic and drug addict, and in doing so, must be taken into account in any clinical and research assessment of mood and behavior. The dictum that alcoholics and drug addicts drink to feel good is not supported by any of the studies other than those that accept the addict's retrospective self-report verbatim.[3] Taking this type or self-report in another illness to its logical conclusion, would be to accept prima face a demented patient's self-report that the year is 1891 and nothing is wrong with his/her memory.[7]

Autonomy of Conditions

The autonomous nature of alcohol and drug addiction is a fundamental point, when accepted, greatly clarifies the role of alcohol and drugs in interactions with other psychiatric disorders. Autonomous for addiction means that alcohol and drug use arises spontaneously, stereotypically, and repetitively without an apparent known cause. In this way, addiction shares a similar status to cancer, essential hypertension and schizophrenia, where conditions arise without a unique precipitant or known cause.

Perhaps the closest natural state to addiction are drives such as hunger, thirst, and sex. These autonomous instincts responsible for survival of the organism are relentless and normally achieve expression. Theoretical implications are that alcohol and drugs become entrained by drive states to become an aberrant "instinct" to use alcohol and drugs similar to hunger, thirst and sex. The neurosubstrate for addiction appears to reside in the limbic system specifically the so called "reinforcement area" in association with the instinctual drives. Addiction may be viewed as a neurological disorder arising with psychiatric and behavioral manifestations similar to other neuropsychiatric conditions such as Huntington's Chorea, Alzheimer's Disease or a seizure disorder.[7]

Self-Medication Hypothesis

The self-medication hypothesis does little to clarify the interactions of alcohol and drug disorders with other psychiatric disorders. Moreover, the self-medication hypothesis is detrimental to the diagnosis and treatment of addictive disorders. Literally, the self-medication hypothesis states that alcohol and drug use and addiction are motivated by and dependent on another "underlying" or "causative" condition or state, and thus alcohol/drug use and addictions are not primary or independent conditions. Examples are that "anxiety" is a reason why alcohol is used as a sedative or "depression" is why cocaine is used as a stimulant. While intuitively appealing, these reasons for alcohol and drug use and addiction are lay explanations that are contradicted by experimental studies and clinical experience in addictive disorders.

Self-medication is largely assumed as a cause of alcohol and drug use in clinical practice and studies of patient reports.[3,8] The opposite effects are found in studies in that alcohol and drug use causes anxiety and depression, and alcoholics and drug addicts use alcohol and drug despite worsening anxiety and depression. While anxious and depressed non-alcoholic people may be relieved acutely by alcohol and drugs, they do not use increased amounts. According to studies, in fact, they are more likely to decrease their consumption of alcohol and drugs perhaps because the pharmacologic sequelae of alcohol and drugs is the production of anxiety and depression. This is reviewed in further detail in other sources.[4,5,6,7]

Addiction as a Source of Psychiatric Symptoms in Abstinence

There is a theoretical neuropathic basis for addictive disorders as a genesis of disturbances in mood during intoxication and abstinence. Addictive disorders and mood regulation appear to originate from the structures in the limbic system, and addictive behaviors (drive states) and mood states appear closely linked to similar neurotransmitter systems. Dopamine is implicated in both mood states and addictive reinforcement behaviors, norepinephrine in mood states and alcohol/drug withdrawal and serotonin in mood states and alcohol consumption. Increases or decreases in these neurotransmitters are associated with increases or decreases in mood states and addictive behaviors.[7]

Of critical relevance to diagnosis and treatment is that anxiety and depressive syndromes arising from addictive disorders do not respond to treatment for traditional psychiatric disorders such as antianxiety, antidepressant, and anti-psychotic medications or psychotherapy. Specific treatment of the addictive disorders as the root cause will often result in amelioration of the anxiety and depression. Correspondingly, attempts at pharmacological intervention for addictive disorders will have a greater likelihood of success if aimed at the addictive processes rather than traditional psychiatric treatment of altered moods and thinking.

The success obtained by millions of recovered alcoholics and drug addicts can attest to validity and reliability of these concepts. Moreover, treatment outcome studies confirm that abstinence rates of greater than 70% can be accomplished in alcoholics and drug addicts through specific treatment of addiction.[9,10] Along with abstinence, there is usually a marked improvement in mood and behavior over time, and often a resolution of severe psychiatric syndromes with specific treatment of addictive diseases.[2,9,10]

GENETICS AND FAMILY HISTORY STUDIES

Most adoption, twin, and high risk studies reveal that alcohol and drug disorders are genetically independent from other psychiatric disorders. In familial studies where overlap of alcohol and drug induced syndromes commonly occurs with other psychiatric disorders, alcohol/drug disorders run independently from other psychiatric disorders. One would expect a genetic and familial relationship if the disorders were dependent on each other or that alcohol and drug disorders were part of the spectrum of psychiatric disorders.[11,12,13]

PREVALENCE RATES IN ADDICTION AND PSYCHIATRIC SETTINGS

The prevalence rates for the co-occurrence of alcohol and drug disorders with other psychiatric disorders differ greatly depending on the population studied, perspective of the examiner, the method of study (retrospective vs prospective) and the length of follow up.[13] If the population is an addiction unit, and the examiner an addictionist who considers addiction as an independent disorder, and the follow up prospective over months and years, the prevalence rates for psychiatric disorder co-occurring with addictive disorders will be low, i.e., no greater than the general population: 3.5% for major depression, 0.67% for panic disorder, 1.4% for obsessive-compulsive disorder, 0.1% for somatization disorder, 0.6% for antisocial personality disorders, for schizophrenia, 1.1%, and for phobias, 6%.[14,15] On the other hand, if the population is psychiatric, the examiner a psychiatrist who is applying the self-medication hypothesis, and the study is retrospective with little or no follow up, then the rates for co-occurrence of psychiatric and addictive disorders will be high, i.e., 50% total or 30% in schizophrenia, 50% in schizoaffective disorders, 25% in bipolar, 84% in antisocial and borderline personality disorders, 30% in major depression, and 28% for anxiety disorders.[16,17]

The task of sorting out which is which, where is where, and when is when, is perplexing and unfortunately one still must make deductions on the basis of what one *thinks* is right so that the information will be meaningful for clinical practice and research. The prevalence rates for psychiatric disorders in addiction populations are relatively clear from studies over the past 30 years, but rates for patients in psychiatric settings have been investigated only recently and require further clarification. Because psychiatric disorders are considerably less common than addictive disorders in the general population, therefore, the overlap between the two disorders should occur infrequently in populations of alcoholics and drug addicts. For example, if the rate for alcoholism is 16% and for schizophrenia is 1% in the general population, then most alcoholics are not schizophrenics. Also, if the rate for major depression is 10% in the general population, then probability for alcoholism occurring together with it as an independent event is 1.6% (16% $\times$ 10%). The discussion can only ensue if the two events are not considered independent, or where alcohol and drug disorders are not provided an independent status. Also, if it is not considered that alcohol and drug disorders produce psychiatric syndromes during the intoxication, withdrawal and abstinent states, the rates for comorbidity will be further inflated. Finally, little evidence currently exists to support the notion that psychiatric disorders produce alcohol and drug disorders.[18]

CURRENT LEVEL OF TRAINING

The best predictor of the future standard level of treatment for dual diagnosis patients is the current type of training. The minimum requirements for training in addictive disorders have not been defined in residency training programs. In fact the current amount of time and resources devoted to training residents in addictive disorders is far short of the magnitude of alcohol and drug problems in psychiatric settings. A quick calculation reveals a prevalence rate of at least 50% for alcohol/drug disorders in psychiatric settings versus 2.8% or one month (above average) out of 48 devoted to training for addictive disorders in psychiatric training programs.[19]

Just how much and how long medical schools have been able to avoid diagnosing and treating addictive disorders indicates yet another example of the persistence of the moral attitude and judgmental approach to addictive diseases and "turf issues" among disciplines. More research will not overcome the lack of acceptance by the medical community, and in particular, the psychiatric specialty in the foreseeable future. The stigma that remains is prohibitive, and the fear by physicians and psychiatrists that they will lose their professional status if they are identified with addiction treatment does not advance the diagnosis and treatment of dual diagnosis patients. At the same time, the addictionist must tread what appears to be perilous waters in an effort to expand their knowledge of interactions between addictive diseases and psychiatric disorders.[20]

SUGGESTIONS FOR NEW CONCEPTS
AND TERMINOLOGY IN DUAL DIAGNOSIS

1. Base concepts and definitions on data, not interpretive assumptions or disproven hypotheses.
2. Develop new concepts and definitions where older psychiatric rationale does not explain clinical observations and research findings.
3. Employ data that confirm the role of addiction in alcohol and drug use for clinical practice and future research.
4. Formulate hypotheses for future research that examine addictive disorders in relation to psychiatric syndromes and disorders and not only psychiatric disorders in relation to addictive disorders.
5. Implement treatment programs utilizing clinically accepted forms of intervention and therapies for addictive disorders in

psychiatric settings and for independent psychiatric disorders in addiction settings.

6. Require psychiatrists and other physicians who treat dual diagnosis patients to have adequate training in both addictive and psychiatric disorders and to demonstrate clinical competence, not only written knowledge in addictive disorders.

REFERENCES

1. Imhoff, JE. Countertransference issues in alcoholism and drug addiction. Psychiatr Ann. 1991;21:296-306.

2. Schuckit, M. Clinical implications of primary diagnostic groups among alcoholics. Arch Gen Psychiatr. 1985;42:1043-1049.

3. Weiss, RD, Griffin, ML, Miris, SM. Drug abuse as self medication for depression. An empirical study. Am J Drug an Alc. Abuse. 1992;18(2):121-130.

4. Mayfield DG. Alcohol and affect. In Goodwin DW, Erickson CK, ed. Experimental studies in alcoholism and affective disorders. New York: SP Medical and Scientific, 1979.

5. Schuckit MA, Irwin M, Brown ST. The history of anxiety symptoms among 171 primary alcoholics. J Stud Alcohol. 1991;51:31-41.

6. Tamerin JS, Mendelson, JH. The psychodynamics of chronic inebriation. Observations of alcoholics during the process of drinking in an experimental group setting. Am J Psychiatr. 1969;125:886.

7. Miller NS, Gold, MS. Dependence syndromes: a critical analysis of essential features. Psychiatr Ann. 1991;21:282-290.

8. Khantzian ES. The self-medication hypothesis of addictive disorders: focus on heroin and cocaine dependence. Am J Psychiatr. 1986;142:1259-64.

9. Miller NS, Millman RB, Keskinen S. Outcome at six and twelve months post-inpatient treatment for cocaine and alcohol dependence. Adv Alcohol Subs Abuse. 1990;9:3/4:101-120.

10. Harrison A, Hoffman NG, Streed SG. Treatment outcome. In: Miller NS, ed. Comprehensive handbook of drug and alcohol addiction. New York: Marcel Dekker Inc, 1991.

11. Schuckit MA. Genetic and clinical implications of alcoholism and affective disorders. Am J Psychiatr. 1986;143:140-147.

12. Schuckit MA, Sweeney S. Substance use and mental health problems among sons of alcoholics and controls. J Stud Alcohol. 1987;48:528-534.

13. Vaillant GE, Milofsky EP. The etiology of alcoholism: a prospective viewpoint. Am Psychol. 1982;37:494-503.

14. Myers JD, Weissman MM, Tischler GL et al. Six-month prevalence of psychiatric disorders in three communities. Arch Gen Psychiatr. 1984;41:959-967.

15 .Schuckit MA. Alcoholism and other psychiatric disorders. Hosp Comm Psychiatr. 1983;34:1022-1027.

16. Regier DA, Farmer ME, Rae DS, et al. Comorbidity of mental disorders with alcohol and other drug abuse. JAMA. 1990;264:19, 2511-2518.

17. Helzer JE, Przybeck TR. The co-occurrence of alcoholism with other psychiatric disorders in the general population and its impact on treatment. J Stud Alcohol. 1988;49:219-224.

18. Miller NS, Gold MS. Alcohol. New York: Plenum Press, 1991.

19. Ries RK, Samson H. Substance abuse among inpatient psychiatric patients: clinical and training issues. Subst Abuse. 1987;3:28-34.

20. Miller NS, Ries RK. Drug and alcohol dependence and psychiatric populations: the need for diagnosis, intervention, and training, Compr Psychiatr. 1991;32:3:268-276.

Genetic and Family Studies in Psychiatric Illness and Alcohol and Drug Dependence

Stephen H. Dinwiddie, MD
Theodore Reich, MD

SUMMARY. The high prevalence of comorbid psychiatric disorders among patients with substance dependence both confuses diagnosis and complicates treatment. One way of separating substance dependence and comorbid conditions is to use the family, rather than the individual, as the unit of study. Results from family, twin, and adoption studies indicate the existence of a heritable and specific liability to alcohol dependence independent of other psychiatric disease, and perhaps to other substance dependence, as well. However, substance dependence, like many other psychiatric disorders, is a clini-

Stephen H. Dinwiddie is Assistant Professor of Psychiatry, Washington University School of Medicine and Jewish Hospital of St. Louis.

Theodore Reich is Professor of Psychiatry and Genetics, Washington University School of Medicine and Jewish Hospital of St. Louis.

This paper was supported by grant number MH46276, AA08401 and AA08403 (Dr. Dinwiddie) and MH46280, MH45522 and MH31302 (Dr. Reich).

Reprint requests should be addressed to Dr. Stephen H. Dinwiddie, Department of Psychiatry, Jewish Hospital of St. Louis, 216 S. Kingshighway, St. Louis, MO 63110.

[Haworth co-indexing entry note]: "Genetic and Family Studies in Psychiatric Illness and Alcohol and Drug Dependence." Dinwiddie, Stephen H., and Theodore Reich. Co-published simultaneously in *Journal of Addictive Diseases,* (The Haworth Press, Inc.) Vol. 12, No. 3, 1993, pp. 17-27; and: *Comorbidity of Addictive and Psychiatric Disorders* (Ed: Norman S. Miller, and Barry Stimmel) The Haworth Press, Inc., 1993, pp. 17-27. Multiple copies of this article/ chapter may be purchased from The Haworth Document Delivery Center. Call 1-800-3-HAWORTH (1-800-342-9678) between 9:00 - 5:00(EST) and ask for DOCUMENT DELIVERY CENTER.

cally and etiologically heterogeneous entity, which both complicates patterns of familial transmission and underlines the need for more precise description of subforms of illness.

Faced with the task of integrating the plethora of studies linking alcohol dependence, other psychoactive substance dependence, and other psychiatric syndromes, one rapidly becomes overwhelmed. Rather than finding a schema with cause always neatly linked to effect (for example conduct difficulties leading to substance experimentation and dependence, leading to further social problems and depression) it soon becomes obvious that the interrelationship between substance dependence, mood disorders, antisocial behavior, and anxiety states is a tangled web of cause and effect, permissive and protective influences, inherited and learned factors.

If the illness to be studied is familial, one way of disentangling the relationship between these conditions is by using the family, rather than the individual, as the unit of study. Thus, while comorbidity is usually thought of as the occurrence of two (or more) diseases in the same individual, either at the same time or on a lifetime basis (lifetime comorbidity), one may also speak of comorbidity within the family, that is, the occurrence of a second illness within the proband's family at a rate above that expected in the population at large. When such familial associations are seen, individuals with the first, the second, and both illnesses may be compared in order to identify possible etiologic factors.

This does not necessarily mean that all cases or even the majority of cases of an illness must be familial, nor does it establish a genetic basis for these illnesses. It simply means that the prevalence of the disorder among relatives of a proband with the disorder is higher than its prevalence in the general population. Once the familial occurrence of an illness is established, study of its inheritance can lead to deeper understanding of its pathogenesis as well as clarifying its relationship to comorbid conditions.

Therefore, the first step is to demonstrate the familial occurrence of the disorder in question. As it happens, familial transmission has been demonstrated in psychiatric illnesses including the affective disorders,[1,2] schizophrenia,[3] antisocial personality disorder,[4] anxiety disorders,[5] Briquet's syndrome,[6] and attention deficit disorder,[7] among others.

Similarly, the familial nature of alcoholism is one of the most solidly-based findings in psychiatry. Despite great diversity in populations selected, diagnostic practices, and research strategies employed, researchers have consistently concluded that the risk of alcoholism is elevated up to seven-fold among first-degree family members of alcoholics.[8,9] While women are less often affected than men (both in the general population and within alcoholic families), there is no sex difference in transmission; that is, relatives have the same degree of risk for alcoholism whether the proband is male or female.[10]

But family studies alone typically only suggest the presence of heritable factors. While the presence of biologically transmissible features may be established based on comparing transmission between various classes of relatives, adoption and twin studies are considered the primary means of separating constitutional and learned determinants of risk for illness. In the case of alcoholism, evidence from both twin and adoption studies also strongly supports the conclusion that heritable, non-environmental factors have substantial influence on risk of illness.[9,11-13]

However, these studies just as strongly demonstrate that like many common, complex diseases (such as juvenile-onset diabetes or hypertension), alcohol dependence does not follow any easily identified pattern of inheritance; its appearance depends on an interaction between inborn, constitutional factors and postnatal exposure and experiences.[14] Moreover, both adoption and twin studies indicate the existence of subforms of alcohol dependency with distinct patterns of inheritance and degree of susceptibility to postnatal influences.[13,15-16]

Consequently, finding a biological marker specific for alcohol dependence would be a significant step forward. In particular, demonstration of linkage between the disease and a known chromosomal site could rapidly lead to precise identification and molecular characterization of a genetic liability factor. Elucidation of the function of the normal allele(s) and finding how the disease-related allele(s) differed could immeasurably advance our understanding of the pathogenesis of alcohol dependence.

While there is evidence to suggest association with a variety of markers,[17,18] recently interest has focused on a possible association with the dopamine D2 receptor, first reported by Blum et al.,[19] who found the A1 allele at that site in 69% of alcoholics, versus 20% of nonalcoholic controls.

Bolos et al.[20] did not replicate their results, instead finding the A1 allele in 38% of alcoholics versus 30% of nonalcoholics, and did not find linkage with the D2 dopamine receptor locus in two families. Next, Parsian et al.[21] found an association between the A1 allele and alcoholism (in 41% of alcoholics versus 12% of controls), with an even more striking difference in that the allele was found in 60% of the severe alcoholics in their sample. However, like Bolos et al., they were unable to demonstrate linkage to the D2 receptor site. Finally, Noble et al.[22] reexamined the specimens reported by Blum et al.[19] and found a progressive decrease in dopamine binding sites among alcoholics as compared to nonalcoholics, with the number lowest in the homozygous A1A1 subjects, suggesting that genotype at the D2 locus, through its expression of receptors, might influence susceptibility to some form of alcoholism.

Research on the inheritance of other forms of drug dependence, as might be expected, is less advanced.[23] While animal studies support the role of genetic factors in alcohol and drug-seeking behavior,[24] demonstration of intergenerational transmission in humans has proven difficult, for several reasons.

First, relative to alcohol dependence, other drug dependence remains relatively rare: In the ECA study, lifetime prevalence of opioid abuse and dependence, for example, was found to be 0.7%, compared to 11-16% for alcohol abuse and dependence.[25,26] Moreover, legal sanctions against drug use and social disapproval tend to make data-gathering and recruitment of subjects more difficult.[27]

Another difficulty is that on a lifetime basis drug users, though they may have specific preferences, tend not to restrict use to one drug or class of drug, thus complicating studies of transmission. As a result, researchers have at times assumed a single underlying spectrum of vulnerability to alcohol and all illicit drugs or grouped illicit drugs together without respect to pharmacologic properties.[14]

Finally, changes in the availability of illicit drugs would be expected to profoundly alter observed patterns of inheritance. Even if in fact genetic factors played a major role in conveying susceptibility to dependence on a given drug (such as cocaine or heroin), without exposure the trait would not be revealed.

Nonetheless, evidence exists to suggest a familial liability to substance abuse and dependence. Meller et al.,[28] using a family history protocol to study 305 probands admitted for substance abuse or dependence, found 97 with alcohol abuse/dependence only, 27 with drug abuse/dependence, and 177 with alcohol plus other substance abuse/dependence. Probands with drug abuse/dependence (amphetamine and cannabis abuse/dependence being the most common) more frequently reported having a family history of drug abuse than probands with alcohol abuse/dependence (18.5% vs. 3%) and also more often reported first-degree relatives with both alcohol and other drug use, 26% as compared to 14%.

Similarly, Rounsaville et al.,[29] using Research Diagnostic Criteria (RDC) to report diagnoses in a large family study of opiate addicts, found high rates of ASP, major depression, alcoholism, and drug abuse among first-degree relatives. Indeed, their study was large enough to allow subdivision of opiate addicts into groups without other RDC diagnoses, opiate addiction plus major depression, or opiate addiction plus ASP. They had difficulty in demonstrating specific intergenerational transmission of opiate use, since only 1% of the parents had used opiates, but their data nonetheless showed familial aggregation of drug abuse, with rates ranging from 17.5% to 22.8% of first-degree relatives, versus 3.3% among relatives of normal controls, corresponding to a 13.7-fold increase in adjusted odds of drug use given a family history of opiate addiction.

A third large family study, by Mirin et al.,[30] evaluated 350 inpatients admitted for drug abuse, of whom slightly over half were opiate users, another 1/3 were cocaine users, and the remainder primarily used sedative-hypnotics. Among first-degree relatives overall, 9.5% had a drug abuse diagnosis. But the rate of drug abuse among relatives differed substantially based on the proband's drug of choice, from 16% of male relatives of cocaine users to 2% of male relatives of sedative-hypnotic users. In contrast, rates of alcoholism among family members were comparable across groups, again suggesting specific aggregation of drug abuse within families.

Thus, despite significant obstacles to such investigations, evidence from three large family studies suggests the familial association of drug dependence. However, there have been few studies which have explicitly tried to separate genetic and environmental factors. The only reported study of twins[13] found that concordance for drug abuse/dependence (by *DSM-III* criteria) was significantly higher in monozygotic than dizygotic male, but not female, twins. However, the MZ/DZ ratio of concordance for abuse and dependence was similar across sex (1.45 for males versus 1.37 for females), suggesting that the negative finding in females was due to lack of statistical power.

An adoption study of 443 adoptees by Cadoret et al.,[31] also suggested heritability of drug dependence, but found that it was related to a biological background of alcohol problems and ASP such that adoptees with drug abuse but not ASP tended to have a biological background of alcohol problems, while a biological background of ASP predicted ASP in the adoptee, which was in turn highly correlated with drug abuse.

FAMILIAL COMORBIDITY
IN SUBSTANCE DEPENDENCE

In sum, it seems clear that alcoholism and other substance dependence aggregate in families. There is strong evidence for the existence of genetic liability for alcoholism, and weaker, though still considerable, support for the role of genetic factors in other substance dependence. However, these factors may differ in their likelihood of causing specific substance dependence or other specific familial psychiatric syndromes.

Perhaps the best studied situation is the familial co-occurrence of alcoholism and depression. Cloninger et al.[32] and Merikangas et al.[33] have concluded that, although these disorders often occur together both in the individual and in their families, the disorders are transmitted separately. Subjects with depression but not alcoholism have an excess of depression, but not alcoholism, in their relatives; those with alcoholism and depression tend to transmit both.

Similarly, based on adoption data, von Knorring et al.[34] found no significant excess of depression among parents of substance abusers as compared to controls (2.5% vs. 4.8%), nor was an excess of treated substance abuse seen in parents of adoptees with affective disorder versus controls (6.3% vs. 3.9%).

There may also be a familial association between alcoholism and certain anxiety syndromes, agoraphobia in particular, with 17% to

26% of relatives of agoraphobics reportedly having alcohol-related difficulties.[35,36] Other anxiety disorders, however, appear to convey less risk for alcoholism,[37] and it is probable that most anxiety symptoms in alcoholics are directly related to heavy drinking, rather than reflecting an independent disorder.[38]

Other major areas of familial comorbidity have proved to be more difficult to address. ASP conveys the highest risk of any disorder for dependence on alcohol or other substances, and family studies of alcohol and drug dependence have consistently found elevated rates of ASP in relatives.[10,29] The association between ASP and problematic alcohol use is so close, in fact, that alcoholism has often been considered to be a part of the syndrome or a complication of ASP rather than necessarily being a distinct entity.[39,40] This view is given some support by Hesselbrock et al.,[41] who found that a family history of ASP powerfully influenced the course of alcoholism, with ASP alcoholics experiencing earlier onset of problems and more psychosocial consequences of drinking. Similarly, Rounsaville et al.[29] found no appreciable difference in rates of ASP among relatives of probands with opiate addiction regardless of any secondary diagnosis the proband had, including ASP. A diagnosis of ASP in the proband conveyed no risk for ASP in the relative in excess of that conveyed by the opiate addiction, possibly indicating substantial overlap between the two conditions.

On the other hand, Cadoret et al.[42] and Cadoret et al.,[43] on the basis of adoption studies, have found evidence of independent genetic inheritance of alcoholism and ASP. Since both ASP and alcoholism are heterogeneous phenotypes,[44,45] this conflict may result from using definitions which are too broad: In order to clarify the familial association (or independence) of these disorders, more homogeneous subgroups of both disorders need to be defined.

On the basis of a large adoption study and subsequent work, Cloninger[46,47] has suggested that at least two more homogeneous subforms of alcoholism exist. Analysis of records on 862 men and 913 women born in Stockholm between 1930 and 1949, of known paternity and adopted by nonrelatives at an early age revealed two patterns of alcohol abuse. Type 1 alcoholics, characterized by later onset of alcohol-related difficulties, benders, guilt over drinking, alcoholic liver disease, and loss of control over drinking, tended to have alcohol abuse, but not criminality, found in their biological parents. Prolonged hospitalization prior to adoption and low socioeconomic status in the adoptive parents appeared to be risk indicators for severity; without such exacerbating factors, course of illness tended to be mild. Daughters of biological fathers with Type 1 background tended to have an increase in alcohol abuse, but not criminality, somatoform disorders, or other psychiatric disorders.

Characteristics of Type 2 alcoholics include early onset of alcohol problems, fighting while intoxicated, auto troubles while drinking, and inability to abstain from alcohol. Their biological fathers tended to have a background of both treatment for alcoholism and of significant criminality; mothers had no excess of either. Regardless of postnatal environment, their adopted-away sons had a ninefold increase in risk of alcohol abuse, yielding an estimate of the heritability of liability to this form of alcohol abuse of 90% in men. Unlike the daughters of Type 1 men, daughters of Type 2 fathers showed no increase in either alcohol abuse or criminality, but did have a significant increase in somatoform disorders.

CONCLUSION

Family studies of substance dependence can help to untangle the complex issue of comorbidity by identifying which illnesses are inherited together and how genetic and environmental factors promote illness or protect against it. On the basis of studies of inheritance, as well as precise clinical description and laboratory measurements, homogeneous subforms of illness may be identified, allowing for more precise characterization of causal mechanisms. Moreover, by identifying heritable factors within the disease phenotype, family, twin and adoption studies can point to specific characteristics which may profitably be evaluated by genetic linkage studies.

Evidence to date suggests that liability to alcoholism has a genetic component, with some forms apparently highly heritable. Most anxiety symptoms in alcoholics appear to be a consequence of heavy drinking, rather than being independent disorders, though there is evidence to suggest independent transmission of agoraphobia. Other cases of alcoholism, particularly those associated with early onset, may also be associated with even earlier onset of criminal or other antisocial behavior, though in such cases adoption studies indicate independent genetic transmission. While depressive symptoms are frequent, for most, depression appears to be separately inherited, suggesting that for many alcoholics, a depressive syndrome is a complication of alcohol dependence, rather than being a second, independent illness. Such findings further underscore the need to separate the phenotype of substance dependence into more clinically distinct subgroups, based on coexistent disorders, laboratory findings, and family history.

REFERENCES

1. Moldin SO, Reich T, Rice JP. Current perspectives on the genetics of unipolar depression. Behav Genet 1991; 21(3):211-42.

2. Rice JP, Reich T, Andreasen NC, Endicott J, Van Eerdewegh M, Fishman R, Hirschfeld RMA, Klerman GL. The familial transmission of bipolar illness. Arch Gen Psychiatry 1987; 44(5):441-447.

3. Rice JP, McGuffin P. Genetic etiology of schizophrenia and affective disorders. In: Cooper AM, Guze SB, Judd L, Klerman GL, Michels R, Cavenar JO, Solnit AJ, eds., *Psychiatry*. Philadelphia, PA: JB Lippincott, 1985:1(62)1-24.

4. Cloninger CR, Reich T, Guze SB. The multifactorial model of disease transmission: II. Sex differences in the familial transmission of sociopathy (antisocial personality). Br J Psychiatry 1975; 127:11-22.

5. Weissman MM. The epidemiology of anxiety disorders: Rates, risks and familial patterns. J Psychiatr Res 1988; 22(Suppl 1):99-114.

6. Cloninger CR, Reich T, Guze SB. The multifactorial model of disease transmission: III. Familial relationship between sociopathy and hysteria (Briquet's syndrome). Br J Psychiatry 1975; 127:23-32.

7. Biederman J, Munir K, Knee D, Habelow W, Armentano M, Autor S, Hoge SK, Waternaux C. A family study of patients with attention deficit disorder and normal controls. J Psychiatr Res 1986; 20(4):263-74.

8. Cotton NS. The familial incidence of alcoholism. J Stud Alc 1979; 40(1):89-116.

9. Merikangas KR. The genetic epidemiology of alcoholism. Psychol Med 1990; 20:11-22.

10. Guze SB, Cloninger CR, Martin R, Clayton PJ. Alcoholism as a medical disorder. Compr Psychiatry 1986; 27(6):501-10.

11. Goodwin DW, Schulsinger F, Lermansen L, Guze SB, Winokur G. Alcohol problems in adoptees raised apart from alcoholic biological parents. Arch Gen Psychiatry 1973; 28(2): 238-43.

12. Cadoret RJ, Cain CA, Grove WM. Development of alcoholism in adoptees raised apart from alcoholic biologic relatives. Arch Gen Psychiatry 1980; 37(5):561-63.

13. Pickens RW, Svikis DS, McGue M, Lykken DT, Heston LL, Clayton PJ. Heterogeneity in the inheritance of alcoholism. Arch Gen Psychiatry 1991;48(1): 19-28.

14. Dinwiddie SH, Cloninger CR. Family and adoption studies in alcoholism and drug addiction. Psychiatric Ann 1991; 21(4):206-14.

15. Cloninger CR, Bohman M, Sigvardsson S. Inheritance of alcohol abuse. Cross-fostering analysis of adopted men. Arch Gen Psychiatry 1981; 38(8):861-8.

16. Bohman M, Sigvardsson S, Cloninger CR. Maternal inheritance of alcohol abuse. Cross-fostering analysis of adopted women. Arch Gen Psychiatry 1981; 38(9):965-69.

17. Hill SY, Goodwin DW, Cadoret R, Osterland CK, Doner SM. Association and linkage between alcoholism and eleven serological markers. J Stud Alc 1975; 36(7):981-92.

18. Hill SY, Aston C, Rabin B. Suggestive evidence of genetic linkage between alcoholism and the MNS blood group. Alc Clin Exp Res 1988; 12(6):811-14.

19. Blum K, Noble EP, Sheridan PJ, Montgomery A, Ritchie T, Jagadeeswaran P, Nogami H, Briggs AH, Cohn JB. Allelic association of human dopamine D2 receptor gene in alcoholism. JAMA 1990; 263(15):2055-60.

20. Bolos AM, Dean M, Lucas-Derse S, Ramsburg M, Brown GL, Goldman D. Population and pedigree studies reveal a lack of association between the dopamine D2 receptor gene and alcoholism. JAMA 1990; 264(24):3156-60.

21. Parsian A, Todd RD, Devor EJ, O'Malley KL, Suarez BK, Reich T, Cloninger CR. Alcoholism and alleles of the human D2 dopamine receptor locus. Arch Gen Psychiatry 1991; 48(7): 655-63.

22. Noble EP, Blum K, Ritchie T, Montgomery A, Sheridan PJ. Allelic association of the D2 dopamine receptor gene with receptor-binding characteristics in alcoholism. Arch Gen Psychiatry 1991; 48(7):648-54.

23. Pickens RW, Svikis DS. Genetic influences in human substance abuse. J Addict Dis 1991; 10(1-2):205-13.

24. Crabbe JC, McSwigan JD, Belknap JK. The role of genetics in substance abuse. In: Galizio M, Maisto SA, eds. *Determinants of Substance Abuse*. New York, NY: Plenum Press, 1985:13-64.

25. Anthony JC, Helzer JE. Syndromes of drug abuse-dependence. In: Robins LE, Regier DA, eds. *Psychiatric Disorders in America*. New York, NY: The Free Press, 1990:116-54.

26. Robins LN, Helzer JE, Weissman MM et al. Lifetime prevalence of specific psychiatric disorders in three sites. Arch Gen Psychiatry 1984; 41(10):949-56.

27. Kozel NJ, Adams EH. Epidemiology of drug abuse: an overview. Science 1989; 234:970-74.

28. Meller WH, Rinehart R, Cadoret RJ, Troughton E. Specific familial transmission in substance abuse. Int J Addict 1988; 23(10):1029-39.

29. Rounsaville BJ, Kosten TR, Weissman MM, Prusoff B, Pauls D, Anton SF, Merikangas K. Psychiatric disorders in relatives of probands with opiate addiction. Arch Gen Psychiatry 1991; 48(1):33-42.

30. Mirin SM, Weiss RD, Griffin ML, Michael JL. Psychopathology in drug abusers and their families. Compr Psychiatry 1991; 32(1):36-51.

31. Cadoret RJ, Troughton E, O'Gorman TW, Heywood E. An adoption study of genetic and environmental factors in drug abuse. Arch Gen Psychiatry 1986;43(12):1131-36.

32. Cloninger CR, Reich T, Wetzel R. Alcoholism and affective disorders: Familial associations and genetic models. In: Goodwin DW, Erickson C, eds., *Alcoholism and the Affective Disorders*. New York, NY, Spectrum Publishing 1979:57-86.

33. Merikangas KR, Leckman JF, Prusoff BA, Pauls DL, Weissman MM. Familial transmission of depression and alcoholism. Arch Gen Psychiatry 1985; 42(4):367-72.

34. von Knorring A-L, Cloninger CR, Bohman M, Sigvardsson S. An adoption study of depressive disorders and substance abuse. Arch Gen Psychiatry 1983; 40(9):943-50.

35. Noyes R, Crowe RR, Harris EL, et al. Relationship between panic disorder and agoraphobia: a family study. Arch Gen Psychiatry 1986; 43:227-32.

36. Munjack KJ, Moss HB. Affective disorder and alcoholism in families of agoraphobics. Arch Gen Psychiatry 1981; 38:869-71.

37. Kushner MG, Sher KJ, Beitman BD. The relation between alcohol problems and the anxiety disorders. Am J Psychiatry 1990;147(6):685-95.

38. Schuckit MA, Irwin M, Brown SA. The history of anxiety symptoms among 171 primary alcoholics. J Stud Alc 1990; 51(1):34-41.

39. Schuckit MA. Alcoholism and sociopathy-diagnostic confusion. Quart J Stud Alc 1973; 34:157-64.

40. Cleckley H. *The Mask of Sanity*. St. Louis, MO, C.V. Mosby Co, 1982.

41. Hesselbrock VM, Hesselbrock MN, Stabenau JR. Alcoholism in men patients subtyped by family history and antisocial personality. J Stud Alc 1985; 46(1): 59-64.

42. Cadoret RJ, O'Gorman TW, Troughton E, Heywood E. Alcoholism and antisocial personality. Arch Gen Psychiatry 1985; 42(2):161-67.

43. Cadoret RJ, Troughton E, O'Gorman TW. Genetic and environmental factors in alcohol abuse and antisocial personality. J Stud Alc 1987; 48(1):1-8.

44. Cloninger CR, Reich T. Genetic heterogeneity in alcoholism and sociopathy. In: Kety SS, Rowland LP, Sidman RL, Matthysse SW, eds, *Genetics of Neurological and Psychiatric Disorders* New York, NY, Raven Press, 1983:145-65.

45. Whitters A, Troughton E, Cadoret RJ, Widmer RB. Evidence for clinical heterogeneity in antisocial alcoholics. Compr Psychiatry 1984; 25(2):158-64.

46. Cloninger CR, Bohman M, Sigvardsson S, von Knorring A-L. Psychopathology in adopted-out children of alcoholics. The Stockholm adoption study. In: Galanter M, ed., *Recent Developments in Alcoholism* 1985; 3:37-51.

47. Cloninger CR. Neurogenetic adaptive mechanisms in alcoholism. Science 1987; 236:410-16.

Hypothesized Neurochemical Models for Psychiatric Syndromes in Alcohol and Drug Dependence

Irl L. Extein, MD
Mark S. Gold, MD

SUMMARY. Exploration of the neurochemistry of psychiatric and substance use disorders in dual diagnosis patients may help explain the greater than chance comorbidity of these disorders and lead to advances in treatment. This paper will focus on the hypothesized neurochemical changes associated with primary substance use disorders which might lead to secondary psychiatric disorders by mimicking the hypothesized neurochemical changes of primary psychiatric disorders. For example, hypothesized serotonergic deficits in alcoholism, endorphin deficits in opioid dependence, and dopamine depletion in cocaine dependence all might predispose to depression. A vicious cycle of cocaine dependence and depression and a vicious cycle of alcohol and drug dependence and panic anxiety are reviewed as models for hypothesized alcohol or drug withdrawal related neurochemical changes predisposing to continued chemical dependency.

Irl L. Extein was Medical Director and Mark S. Gold, Director of Research, Lake Hospital of the Palm Beaches, Lake Worth, FL.

Reprint requests should be addressed to Irl L. Extein, 1050 N.W. 15th Street, Suite 115, Boca Raton, FL 33486.

[Haworth co-indexing entry note]: "Hypothesized Neurochemical Models for Psychiatric Syndromes in Alcohol and Drug Dependence." Extein, Irl L., and Mark S. Gold. Co-published simultaneously in *Journal of Addictive Diseases,* (The Haworth Press, Inc.) Vol. 12, No. 3, 1993, pp. 29-43; and: *Comorbidity of Addictive and Psychiatric Disorders* (Ed: Norman S. Miller, and Barry Stimmel) The Haworth Press, Inc., 1993, pp. 29-43. Multiple copies of this article/chapter may be purchased from The Haworth Document Delivery Center. Call 1-800-3-HAWORTH (1-800-342-9678) between 9:00 - 5:00(EST) and ask for DOCUMENT DELIVERY CENTER.

Exploration of the neurochemistry of dual diagnosis patients reinforces the need for treatment approaches that take into account both aspects of illness.

INTRODUCTION

The prevalence and clinical significance of patients with dual psychiatric and substance use disorders has been recognized only in the last several years.[1-4] Epidemiological studies of such dual diagnosis patients show that the comorbidity is significantly above chance. Defining primary in terms of chronology, 29% of patients with a primary psychiatric disorders had a secondary substance use disorder; 37% of primary alcoholic patients had a secondary psychiatric disorder; and 53% of patients with drug abuse or dependence had a secondary psychiatric disorder.[5] Dual diagnosis patients can present challenges in treatment. Clinical experience suggests that unless both aspects of the problem are addressed, treatment of either one is unlikely to be successful. Total sobriety and abstinence from drugs of abuse must be the initial focus of treatment, with involvement in Twelve-Step programs. Major psychiatric syndromes present post-detoxification need to be treated.

In the last three or four decades our understanding of the neurochemistry of psychiatric disorders and substance use disorders has grown. However, extensive neurochemical research focused on dual diagnosis patients is limited. Inquiry into the neurochemistry of dual diagnosis needs to involve integrating both aspects neurochemically and will no doubt lead to a better understanding of the prevalence of comorbidity and better and more specific forms of treatment. Inquiry into the neurochemistry of dual diagnosis patients would hope to identify what is special about their neurochemistry, not simply the neurochemistry of psychiatric disorders added to the neurochemistry of substance use disorders. However, as a starting place, one would want to consider the neurochemical implications of comorbid disorders from what is known about each separately.

Specific neurochemical abnormalities have been hypothesized for most of the major psychiatric state disorders including mania, major depressive disorders, schizophrenia and related psychotic states, specific anxiety disorders such as panic disorder and obsessive compulsive disorder, aggressive and other disinhibited states, and a variety of organic mental disorders.[6] In addition, neurochemical changes associated with states of intoxication, withdrawal and chronic use syndromes have been hypothesized for alcohol and a number of major drugs of abuse.[6,7] Clinical genetic studies have identified powerful genetic factors for bipolar disorder, depressive disorder, schizophrenia and alcoholism. Since both psychiatric and substance use disorders tend to be recurrent with episodic acute exacerbations, neurochemical explanations need to take into account the course of the illness and not just single episodes. In this chapter we will explore how the proposed neurochemistry of psychiatric disorders and substance use disorders might interact and relate to each other in individual patients.

There are many hypotheses for the high rates of comorbidity of substance use and psychiatric disorders. Because both types of disorders are common, a significant rate of comorbidity can be attributed simply to chance association. In addition, primary substance use disorders may lead to psychiatric problems on both a psychosocial and neurochemical basis. States of intoxication and withdrawal can produce psychiatric symptoms. The concept of secondary substance abuse has not been proven, [8,9] and can sometimes be used by patients as an excuse to continue substance abuse. The concept of primary and secondary disorders as defined by chronology has limitations. What is considered primary in terms of chronology may not be primary in terms of causality, intensity or clinical focus. Many dual diagnosis patients may best be conceptualized simply as having co-existing disorders, both of which need treatment.

I. The Neurochemistry of Psychiatric Disorders

The neurochemistry of mood disorders has been extensively studied since the 1950's.[6,10] Biological theories of the pathophysiology of depression and manic depressive disorder have focused on the brain monoamine neurotransmitters serotonin (5HT), norepinephrine (NE), and dopamine (DA). The anatomy of these neurochemical systems, with midbrain nuclei projecting to cortex, limbic system and hypothalamus is consistent with the vegetative and cognitive symptomology of depressive disorders. These monoamine neurotransmitter systems are thought to be involved in the regulation of pleasure and reward mechanisms in the brain.[6,7,11] The monoamine theory of depression hypothesized that underactivity in neurotransmission at monoaminergic synapses is associated with depressed states. These changes may be related to decreased neurotransmitter turnover or decreases in receptor sensitivity. A number of associated neurochemical and neuroendocrine changes have been identified. The neurochemical model for depression is essentially a deficit state (see Table 1). This hypothesis is supported by psychopharmacological response studies which showed that essentially all effective antidepressant medications facilitate monoaminergic neurotransmission in the brain by a variety of different mechanisms.[6,10] Mania has been hypothesized to be related to increased activity in brain NE and DA systems.[6,10]

The dopamine hypotheses of schizophrenic psychosis has implicated dopamine systems as critical to the pathophysiology of acute psychotic disorders.[6] A number of neurochemical studies and pharmacological response studies are consistent with this hypothesis. All available antipsychotic agents are DA receptor blockers with the potency of DA blockade highly correlated with clinical antipsychotic potency. The negative symptoms of chronic schizophrenia have been hypothesized to be associated with neurochemical deficits.

No single unified neurochemical theory of anxiety has been developed, though over-activity in NE systems in brain may be involved in the central and sympathetic arousal common to many anxiety

TABLE 1

HYPOTHESIZED DRUG-INDUCED   DEFICIENCY

STATES ASSOCIATED WITH DEPRESSION

Drug	neurochemical deficiency	Mechanism
Opioids (Methadone)	Endogenous opiates	Feedback inhibition of synthesis and receptor down-regulation secondary to chronic use of exogenous opioid agonists
Cocaine	Dopamine	Feedback inhibition of synthesis and depletion of neuronal dopamine secondary to blockade of reuptake of synaptic dopamine
Alcohol	Serotonin	Serotonin depletion

states.[6] Based partly on the response to serotonergic antidepressants such as clomipramine and fluoxetine, a 5HT deficit state has been hypothesized for obsessive compulsive disorder. Studies of panic disorder have shown that specific physiological stimuli such as lactate infusion and carbon dioxide inhalation can trigger episodes of panic disorder in patients with a history of this disorder, and support the notion that this is a specific neurochemical disorder. Identification of the benzodiazepine receptor complex in the brain has suggested possible neurochemical mechanisms for anxiety such as changes in endogenous benzodiazepine ligands or antagonists.

Aggressive behavior and related states of behavioral disinhibition are quite heterogeneous in cause and in neurochemistry.[6] Impulse control disorders can be related to deficits in a variety of neurochemical inhibiting systems and in organic brain syndromes of a variety of origins. However, a specific association between decreased 5HT function and aggressive behavior has been a consistent finding in a number of biochemical studies including studies of the 5HT metabolite 5-hydroxyindoleacetic acid (5HIAA) in cerebro-spinal fluid (CSF). Violent aggression and suicide have been associated with low 5HIAA.[10,12] Thus deficiencies in the neuromodulating effects of 5HT may be associated with aggressive behavior towards self and others.

II. The Neurochemistry of Psychiatric Disorders Secondary to Substance Use Disorders

Neurochemical changes hypothesized to be associated with primary substance abuse problems might mimic the hypothesized neurochemical changes of psychiatric disorders and produce psychiatric syndromes. Cocaine is thought to exert its mood effects by influencing dopaminergic neurotransmission in the brain, though it has some effects on NE and 5HT systems as well.[6,7,11,13] Behavioral effects of cocaine in animals require anatomically intact DA systems in brain. Dopaminergic mesolimbic and mesocortical neuronal systems in the brain have been related to reward or pleasure functions. Cocaine's effects can be blocked by specific DA blockers such as haloperidol. Cocaine seems to exert its acute euphoric effect by blocking the synaptic reuptake of DA and increasing available DA at dopaminergic synapses in the brain. Paranoia is a common complication of cocaine use, usually time limited. Cocaine is thought to precipitate psychosis by stimulating DA neurotransmission. By similar mechanisms cocaine may be related to aggressive behavior also. Panic attacks triggered by cocaine have been described also.[4]

Chronic use of cocaine has been hypothesized to lead to dopamine depletion.[13,14] This proposed dopamine deficiency state may become manifest with chronic use and/or withdrawal, and this is associated clinically with low energy, depression, and intense cocaine craving.[7] Neurochemical findings support this dopamine depletion hypothesis, including the finding of decreased brain DA levels in cocaine dependent rats, decreased serum levels of the DA metabolite homovanilic acid (HVA) and elevated serum levels of prolactin in cocaine dependent patients, and receptor supersensitivity.[13] This dopamine depletion may on a neurochemical basis account for the finding of clinically significant secondary depression in many cocaine addicts, predisposing to continued cocaine dependence (see Figure 1). Studies showed that about one-third of cocaine dependent patients meet criteria for major depressive disorder after detoxification.[2,3] The dopamine depletion hypothesis is also supported by the efficacy of pharmacological agents that have dopamine agonist properties, including bromocriptine and amantadine, in relieving the low energy, depression, and craving associated with cocaine withdrawal.[13,14] The tricyclic antidepressant desipramine has been reported to help maintain abstinence in cocaine addicts by relieving craving and depression.[15] It is interesting to note that though desipramine is thought to have mainly noradrenergic effects, it may have effects on DA systems as well. Desipramine reportedly decreases DA auto-receptor sensitivity, and by decreasing this inhibitory influence increases dopaminergic activity in the brain.[6]

Cocaine kindling may serve as a useful neurochemical model for a variety of psychiatric difficulties.[16] Kindling refers to a phenomenon in which progressively less intense stimulation is required to produce the same effect. This is essentially the physiological opposite of tolerance. As originally described, progressively less intense electrical stimulation is required to kindle a seizure. Cocaine is an epileptogenic substance, and progressively smaller dosages of cocaine are require to produce seizures in animal models. This neurochemi-

FIGURE 1

THE VICIOUS CYCLE OF COCAINE DEPENDENCE AND DEPRESSION

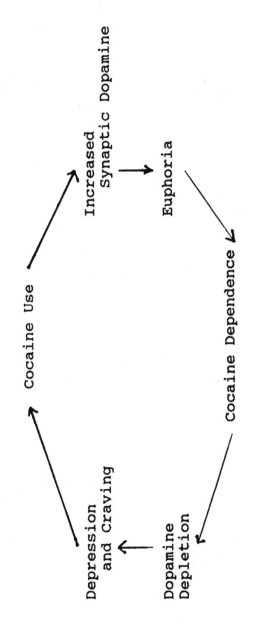

cal property of cocaine might explain increasing psychiatric problems as cocaine dependence progresses, including mood changes, aggression and psychosis. Kindling has also been used as a model for rapid mood cycles. Cocaine kindling has led in part to trials of the anti convulsant carbamazepine in cocaine dependent patients, with some positive preliminary results.[17]

There has been some progress in recent years toward an understanding of the neurochemistry of alcoholism.[6,7,18] Studies suggest that alcohol affects alcoholics differently from non-alcoholics both neurochemically and subjectively. Alcohol produces some of its physiological effects by relatively nonspecific effects on membrane lipid structures with descending effects on central nervous system function as dosage and blood level increase. Specific serotonergic effects of alcohol have been identified as well. Alcohol preferring and alcohol nonpreferring strains of rats differ in 5HT levels in brain. Initially alcohol is thought to augment 5HT functioning with increased CSF levels of 5HIAA reported. This augmentation of 5HT function probably accounts for the initial euphoric effects of alcohol. However, chronic alcohol use reportedly leads to decreased serotoninergic function as identified by decreased CSF 5HIAA levels.[18] This may be the neurochemical substrate for depression, suicidal behavior, and aggression seen in chronic alcoholism. The depression is often associated with active drinking and usually remits with sobriety. One study showed that only 7% of detoxified alcoholics met criteria for major depressive disorder.[3] Decreased 5HT functioning may theoretically predispose to obsessive compulsive symptomatology as well. Zimelidine, a specific 5HT reuptake blocker, has been shown in a preliminary clinical study to decrease alcohol intake in alcoholics.[19] Fluoxetine, which has similar 5HT reuptake blocking effects, has been suggested as an antidepressant that may have specific benefits in alcoholics because of its augmentation of 5HT functioning.

Alcohol, benzodiazepines, and barbiturates affect the brain GABA-benzodiazepine-barbiturate receptor coupled to the chloride channel complex.[6,7] Effects on this endogenous system could lead to sedation, anxiety or behavioral disinhibition and hence predispose to a variety of psychiatric disorders. NE as well as 5HT play important roles in the development of tolerance to alcohol.[6,7] Withdrawal from alcohol and sedatives may be a trigger for the development of panic and other anxiety disorders due to rebound activity in neurochemical systems affected by these substances, including brain NE systems,[4] predisposing to continued alcohol dependence (see Figure 2). Several studies have documented the overlap of alcohol withdrawal and panic symptomatology. However, in patients with a history of panic disorder lactate infusion precipitates panic attacks only in those without a history of alcoholism, suggesting that the neurochemistry of panic disorder secondary to alcoholism may be different from that of primary panic disorder.[20]

Acute alcohol intoxication causes cortical and hence behavioral disinhibition, sometimes leading to aggression and violent behavior.[7] Chronic use can lead to irreversible neuronal damage with cortical atrophy and dementia.[7]

Type II alcoholism is defined by younger age of onset, antisocial and other aggressive behaviors and a thrill-seeking style.[21] The common characteristics of bipolar patients in the hypomanic or manic states and Type II alcoholics, the more than chance association of bipolar disorder with Type II alcoholism, as well as the hypothesized involvement of monoamines in the pathophysiology of both alcoholism and bipolar disorder has led Goodwin to propose an intriguing hypothesis linking Type II alcoholism and bipolar disorder.[10]

The specific mechanisms of marijuana effects on mood, thinking and behavior are not clear. Acute marijuana use can be associated with paranoia, perceptual distortions, panic attacks, and aggressive behavior.[4,7,21] The hallucinogen LSD is an agonist for presynaptic inhibitory 5HT receptors and has direct post-synaptic inhibitory effects in brain serotonergic synapses.[7] Acute effects of LSD and other hallucinogens can lead to psychotic episodes. Flash-backs occur even with prolonged abstinence, possibly related to long-lasting changes in 5HT neurons. Long term repeated use of marijuana, LSD and other hallucinogens can be associated with a "burn out" syndrome of apathy, depression and intellectual deterioration.[4,7]

Endogenous opioids (endorphins and enkephalins) are thought to play a role in modulating mood, pain perception, and stress responses.[6,7] Studies have not confirmed specific endogenous opioid mechanisms in the pathophysiology of major psychiatric illnesses.

FIGURE 2

THE VICIOUS CYCLE OF ALCOHOL AND DRUG DEPENDENCE

AND PANIC ANXIETY

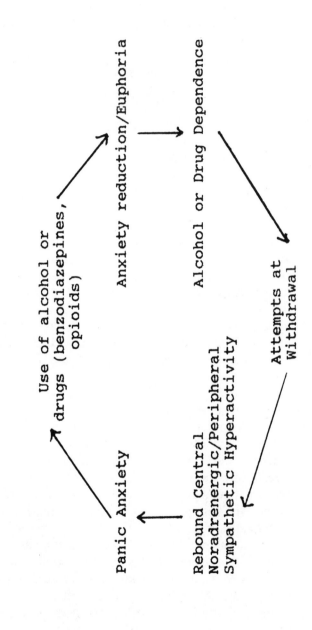

For example, trials of opioid agonist and antagonist drugs in depression and mania have failed to show significant effects.[10] Dependence on opioids would be expected to be associated with feedback suppression of endogenous opioid function. After detoxification these endogenous opioid systems may or may not return to normal. Physiological as well as clinical studies with methadone dependent patients show that in many patients return to normal brain physiology is quite slow.[7] This would be analogous to the decreased adrenal production of corticosteroids in patients treated with high doses of corticosteroids for a prolonged period of time. The chronic abstinence syndrome described following detoxification from opioids may be related to prolonged endogenous opioid deficiencies. This may be the physiological substrate of the depression common in detoxified opioid addicts. Neurochemical changes may be expected to be more pronounced in patients dependent on methadone, with its 24 hour half-life, compared to patients dependent on heroin or other short half-life opioids because of continued receptor stimulation from methadone compared to the "on and off" pattern with heroin use. This may explain why in one study 62% of methadone dependent patients and only 25% of heroin dependent patients were reported to meet criteria for major depressive disorder after detoxification.[3] Major depressive disorders in such patients may represent deficiency states in endogenous opioid systems and may represent organic mood disorders. Studies of the efficacy of antidepressants in detoxified opioid addicts have had mixed results.[3] Pharmacological strategies for opioid abstinence that do not involve maintenance with agonists like methadone, such as the use of the opioid antagonist naltrexone,[7] may be less likely to be associated with deficiencies in endogenous opioid systems and may be less likely to predispose to depression.

Opioids have a direct inhibitory effect on NE systems in brain.[22,23] Thus use of the drugs themselves may predispose to depression. Withdrawal from opioids is associated with acute rebound hyperactivity of brain NE neurons hypothesized to be associated with anxiety, panic, and sometimes violent behavior.[22,23] Electrical and pharmacological stimulation of the noradrenergic nucleus locus ceruleus in primates has been used as an animal model for anxiety and appears very similar to opioid withdrawal in primates. Understanding of the interaction between opioids and NE systems and the neurochemistry of withdrawal has led to the successful treatment of opioid withdrawal with clonidine, an alpha-2 adrenergic agonist which inhibits the locus ceruleus by stimulating pre-synaptic inhibitory receptors.[22]

III. Neurochemical Effects of Substance Abuse in Primary Psychiatric Patients

Secondary abuse of cocaine and other stimulants can be particularly pernicious because of the dual tendencies to exacerbate psychosis and aggression with acute use based on hypothesized facilitation of DA neurotransmission, and to exacerbate depression with chronic use based on hypothesized depletion of brain DA.[13,14] This can be a lethal mix where suicidal tendencies may already exist. Cocaine can exacerbate or precipitate episodes of schizophrenic psychosis, paranoid disorders and other psychotic illnesses, panic disorder, and mania in patients with these disorders.[7,10] Cocaine use by ADHD patients may lead to abuse and dependence with exacerbation of behavioral problems and aggression.

Though alcohol is hypothesized to stimulate 5HT function initially, research into the pathophysiology of chronic alcoholism has noted an association with decreased 5HT functioning in brain and decreased CSF-5HIAA levels.[6,7,10,18] One might speculate that alcoholism in a patient with a depressive disorder may exacerbate depression and suicidal tendencies by compromising 5HT functioning and perpetuate a vicious cycle of further drinking to try to stimulate 5HT pleasure and reward mechanisms which further worsens the 5HT deficits. Alcohol and sedative related cortical suppression can lead to behavioral disinhibition and exacerbate aggressive tendencies. Chronic alcoholism with related decreased 5HT functioning may contribute to aggressive behavior also.

Withdrawal from alcohol and sedatives leads to a state of sympathetic nervous system arousal and possibly increased catecholamine (NE, DA) metabolism in brain as proposed rebound phenomena.[6,7] Withdrawal may also be associated with rebound changes in endogenous benzodiazepine systems[6] as well. These may explain the clinical finding that withdrawal may exacerbate anxiety states such as panic disorder.[4] Some patients with anxiety disorders who develop a secondary alcohol or benzodiazephine dependence may have a particularly difficult time getting off the alcohol or benzodiazepines because of withdrawal-related changes. Often a protracted and well supervised detoxification is needed to avoid exacerbation of anxiety and further dependence on alcohol and sedatives.[4,7] Alprazolam, being an intermediate half-life benzodiazepine,[7] is associated with significant withdrawal symptomatology that may mimic the initial panic symptomology for which the drug was prescribed in the first place.

Anhedonia associated with chronic marijuana use in some patients may exacerbate depressive symptoms and the negative symptoms of schizophrenia. Paranoia and perceptual distortions induced by marijuana may exacerbate schizophrenic and other psychotic illnesses.[5,7] The specific neurochemistry of these effects of marijuana is not well understood.[7] Hallucinogens such as LSD may exacerbate primary psychotic disorders. LSD is thought to exert its effects at least in part by inhibition by central 5HT functioning.[7] Symptoms of withdrawal from opioids have been hypothesized to be related to rebound hyperactivity in brain catecholamine systems, which may explain reports of exacerbation of panic and other anxiety disorders.[7,23] Pain syndromes, which may in some cases have led to opioid narcotic abuse and dependence, might be exacerbated by drug withdrawal with hypothesized deficits in endogenous opioid systems and lead to relapse into opioid abuse, again setting up a vicious cycle.[7]

IV. Psychotropic Medications

The uses of antidepressants in dual diagnosis patients have been discussed. Although lithium can be effective in treating bipolar disorder in cocaine abusers studies have failed to show long-term benefits in cocaine patients without diagnosed bipolar disorder.[15] Early reports had suggested that lithium may help alcoholics maintain sobriety but more recent studies have failed to confirm this finding.[24] Antipsychotic medications partially block the effects of cocaine, consistent with their DA blocking properties.[13] Though antipsychotics may have a place in treating cocaine-related psychosis and aggression, the sedation, dysphoria and extrapyramidal side effects of antipsychotic medications as well as the risk of tardive dyskinesia make antipsychotic medications an unacceptable maintenance treatment for cocaine use disorders. Substance abuse is not uncommon in schizophrenic populations[5,7] and can exacerbate the original psychotic process as well as be a significant factor in noncompliance with prescribed medication. Benzodiazepines are best avoided in dual diagnosis patients because of abuse potential.[4,7]

Other medications with efficacy in anxiety disorders, including beta blockers, antidepressants, and buspirone do not cause euphoria and are not associated with abuse.[6]

REFERENCES

1. Rounsaville BJ, Weissman MM, Kleber H, Wilber C.Heterogeneity of psychiatric diagnosis in treated opiate addicts. Arch Gen Psychiatry 1982; 39:161-66.

2. Mirin SM, Weiss RD, Sollogub A, Michael J. Affective illness in substance abusers. In Mirin SM, ed. Substance Abuse and Psychopathology. Washington, DC:American Psychiatric Press, 1984: 57-77.

3. Extein I, Dackis CA, Gold MS, Pottash ALC. Depression in drug addicts and alcoholics. In: Extein I, Gold MS, eds. Medical Mimics of Psychiatric Disorders. Washington, DC: American Psychiatric Press, Inc., 1986:133- 162.

4. Gold MS, Slaby AE, eds. Dual Diagnosis in Substance Abuse. New York: Marcel Dekker, Inc., 1991.

5. Regier DA, Farmer ME, Rae DS, Locke BZ, Keith SJ, Judd LL, Goodwin FK. Comorbidity of mental disorders with alcohol and drug abuse. JAMA 1990; 264:2511-2518.

6. Meltzer HY, eds. Psychopharmacology: The Third Generation of Progress. New York: Raven Press, 1987.

7. Jaffe, JH. Drug addiction and drug abuse. In: Gilman AG, Rall TW, Mies AS, Taylor P, eds. The Pharmacological Basis of Therapeutics. New York: Pergamon Press, 1990.

8. Hesselbrock MN, Meyer RE, Keener JJ. Psychopathology in hospitalized alcoholics. Arch Gen Psychiatry 1985; 42: 1050-1055.

9. Miller NS, Mahler JC, Belkin BM, FOld MS. Psychiatric diagnosis in alcohol and drug dependence. Annals of Clinical Psychiatry 1991:3:79-89.

10. Goodwin FK, Jamison KR. Manic-Depressive Illness. New York and Oxford: Oxford University Press, 1990.

11. Wise R. The neurobiology of craving: implications for the understanding and treatment of addiction. J. Abnorm Psychol 1988; 118-132.

12. Brown GL, Goodwin FK. Cerebrospinal fluid correlates of suicide attempts and aggression. Ann NY Acad Sci 1986; 487:175-188.

13. Extein I, Dackis CA. Brain mechanisms in cocaine dependency. In: Washton AM, Gold MS eds. New York: The Guilford Press, 1987; 73-84.

14. Dackis CA, Gold MS. Bromocriptine as treatment of cocaine abuse. Lancet 1985; 1:1151-1152.

15. Gawin FH, Kleber HD. Desipramine facilitation of initial cocaine abstinence. Arch Gen Psychiat 1989;46:117- 121.

16. Post RM, Kopanda RT. Cocaine, kindling, and psychosis. Am J Psychiatry 1976; 133:627-634.

17. Halikas JA, Crosby RD, Carlson GA, Crea F,Graves NM, Bowers LD. Cocaine reduction in unmotivated crack users using carbamazepine versus placebo in a short term, double blind crossover design. Clin Parmacol Ther 191;50:81-95.

18. Ballenger JC, Goodwin FK, Major LF, Brown GL. Alcohol and central serotonin metabolism in man. Arch Gen Psychiatry 1979;36:224-227.

19. Naranjo CA, Sellers EM, Roach CA, Woodley DV, Sanchez-Craig M. Sykora K. Zimelidine-induced variations in alcohol intake by nondepressed heavy drinkers. Clin Pharmacol Ther 1984; 35:374-381.

20. George DT, Nutt DJ, Waxman RP, Linnoila M. Panic response to lactate administration in alcoholic and non-alcoholic patients with panic disorders. Am J Psychiatry 1989; 146:1161-1165.

21. Cloninger CR, Dinwiddie SH, Reich T. Epidemiology and genetics of alcoholism. annual Review of Psychiatry 1989; 8:331-346.

22. Gold MS, Redmond DE Jr, Kleber HD. Noradrenergic hyperactivity in opiate withdrawal supported by clonidine reversal of opiate withdrawal. Am J Psychiatry 1979; 136:100-102.

23. Gold MS, Pottash ALC, Sweeney DR, Kleber HD, Redmond DE Jr. Rapid opiate detoxification: Clinical evidence of antidepressant and antipanic effects of opiates. Am J Psychiatry 1979; 136:982-983.

24. Dorus W, Ostrow DG, Anton R, Cushman P, Collins JF, Schaefer M, Charles HL, Desai P, Hayashida M, Malkerneker U, Willenbring M, Fiscella R, Sather MR. Lithium treatment of depressed and nondepressed alcoholics. JAMA 1989; 262:1646-1652.

The Epidemiology of the Comorbidity of Psychiatric and Addictive Disorders: A Critical Review

Valerie D. Raskin, MD
Norman S. Miller, MD

SUMMARY. Assessing the prevalence of the comorbidity of psychiatric and addictive disease using epidemiologic methods results in artifactually high rates. Use of a clinical sample will yield falsely high rates, because substance use is associated with exacerbation of mental illness. Cross sectional design will inflate rates of psychiatric comorbidity in addicts, who attribute substance use to psychological symptoms until well into recovery. Application of exclusionary criteria for independent diagnosis is subject to investigator bias, particularly about the unproven yet popular "self-medication" hypothesis. The psychiatric symptoms which are common in active addiction generally clear within weeks to months of treatment for addiction but

---

Valerie D. Raskin is Assistant Professor of Psychiatry, University of Illinois at Chicago, Chicago, IL.

Norman S. Miller is Associate Professor of Psychiatry, University of Illinois at Chicago, Chicago, IL.

Correspondence should be addressed to Valerie D. Raskin, MD, University of Illinois at Chicago, Department of Psychiatry, 912 S. Wood Street (m/c 913), Chicago, IL 60612.

[Haworth co-indexing entry note]: "The Epidemiology of the Comorbidity of Psychiatric and Addictive Disorders: A Critical Review." Raskin, Valerie D., and Norman S. Miller. Co-published simultaneously in *Journal of Addictive Diseases,* (The Haworth Press, Inc.) Vol. 12, No. 3, 1993, pp. 45-57; and: *Comorbidity of Addictive and Psychiatric Disorders* (Ed: Norman S. Miller, and Barry Stimmel) The Haworth Press, Inc., 1993, pp. 45-57. Multiple copies of this article/chapter may be purchased from The Haworth Document Delivery Center. Call 1-800-3-HAWORTH (1-800-342-9678) between 9:00 - 5:00(EST) and ask for DOCUMENT DELIVERY CENTER.

do not respond to standard psychopharmacologic treatment for primary mental illness. When lengthy follow up periods are employed, substance induced psychiatric syndromes typically resolve. We conclude that while patients treated in psychiatric settings often have comorbid and independent addictive illness, patients treated in addiction settings uncommonly have comorbid psychiatric illness despite common psychiatric symptoms.

Epidemiologic "truth" is subject to many influences. The (1) population sampled, (2) method of design, (3) biases of the examiner, (4) length of study, and (5) treatment intervention are key factors that determine the results from the outset. Prevalence rates vary widely for comorbidity of psychiatric and addictive disorders. Much of the striking discrepancy of epidemiologic data is attributable to who is doing the study, where the study is conducted, and what is being studied.[1]

The term "comorbidity" itself implies the presence of two distinct disorders, psychiatric illness and addiction. The distinction between whether these illnesses merely coincide, are associated syndromes, or are primary vs. secondary remains a debated yet crucial issue. This paper critically reviews epidemiologic findings on comorbidity, examining the influence that each of the above five factors has on epidemiologically derived knowledge about comorbidity. We illustrate how each of these factors contributes to confusion about comorbidity of psychiatric and addictive illness. After examination of the data in light of these factors we conclude that (1) patients in psychiatric settings commonly have comorbid and independent addictive disorder (2) patients in addiction settings uncommonly have comorbid psychiatric illness despite common psychiatric symptoms.

POPULATION SAMPLED

Subjects are either derived from clinical or nonclinical samples. Clinical samples may be further divided into inpatient vs. outpatient, public vs. private, and addiction vs. psychiatry treatment settings. There have been adequate numbers of studies done in each to provide an analysis of the influence of the sampled population on epidemiologic data.

Clinical populations yield higher comorbidity rates than the general population. To the extent that individuals with multiple disorders are more disabled or distressed, such individuals tend to seek treatment; thus comorbid patients will be over represented in clinical samples. In clinical settings, the rate for a particular disorder reflects the treatment provided at the site. For example, a general psychiatric setting will contain higher rates of chronically mentally ill patients because of orientation of the clinicians. Prevalence rates for comorbidity are higher for inpatient vs. outpatient treatment settings, greater for public vs. private settings, and for reimbursement driven diagnoses where one disorder is reimbursed but not another.

Combining these variables, the overall prevalence rate in clinical psychiatric populations for addiction is 50%. In other words, a psychiatric patient has a one in two likelihood of having an addictive disorder. The prevalence rates for addictive disorders vary widely when further broken down into specific psychiatric diagnosis, as indicated in Table 1, column 1.[2-5]

On the other hand, studies reveal that the prevalence rates for psychiatric disorders in clinical populations derived from addiction treatment facilities are considerably lower and typically the same as those found in the general population. These have been relatively well documented in addiction populations accordingly, and are found in the second column of Table 1.[6,7]

The last column in Table 1 further indicates the ratios that these dramatically different rates yield when diagnosis is compared for comorbidity in both settings. As a way of looking at the striking differences, the ratios of the prevalence rates for psychiatric settings to addiction settings have been calculated. While at first surprising, these ratios provide insight into the reason why psychiatric disorders are found so commonly among addictive disorders in some reports. For example, using the ratio for comorbidity for Bipolar Affective Disorder to illustrate how different epidemiologic truth will appear depending on site, one sees that a psychiatric clinician would conclude that Bipolar Affective Disorder is commonly associated with addiction. However, a clinician working in an addiction setting would conclude that addiction is rarely associated with Bipolar Affective Disorder.

TABLE 1: RATIOS OF COMORBITY PREVALENCE RATES COMPARED BY SETTING

DIAGNOSIS: COMORBIDITY	PREVALENCE RATE: PSYCHIATRY SETTING [a]	PREVALENCE RATE: ADDICTION SETTING [b]	RATIO PSYCHIATRY SETTING TO ADDICTION SETTING
Depressive Disorder	30	5	7.5
Bipolar Disorder	50	0.8	62.5
Schizophrenia	50	1.1	27.3
Antisocial Personality Disorder	80	0.6	133.3
Anxiety Disorder	30	3	15
Phobic Disorder	23	6	38.3

a: per cent of patients diagnosed with comorbid addictive disorder

b: per cent of patients diagnosed with comorbid psychiatric disorder

Public community mental health population samples have markedly more chronic mentally ill patients than the private treatment sector. Public psychiatric samples yield the following prevalence rates for comorbid addictive diagnoses: 30% for schizophrenia, 50% for schizoaffective disorders, 30% for affective disorders, and 35% for personality disorders. The rates in outpatient private psychiatric settings are not as well documented but appear to contain lower rates for comorbidity among the chronically mentally ill. Again, to the extent that comorbidity causes greater disability, this may reflect downward socioeconomic drift to public treatment settings.[8-12]

High rates of addictive comorbidity are recognized in the young adult chronic patient, in whom substance dependence is inversely correlated with age. Initial data derived from psychiatric inpatients suggested that as a group, schizophrenic patients preferred psychotomimetics and stimulants but not depressants. This fuelled speculation that the substance used by the young adult chronic patient is selected to self-medicate psychiatric symptoms. However, community based studies indicate that the young adult chronic patient by far most commonly uses those substances most commonly used by nonmentally ill age peers: alcohol and marijuana. Further, when asked, nearly 70% of schizophrenic patients acknowledge using drugs or alcohol for the same reason their age peers report: "to get high." Emergency room samples and community based studies strongly support the finding that drug and alcohol use–even mild use–destabilize the young chronic mentally ill patient and increase the likelihood of hospitalization. Comorbid young chronic mentally ill individuals are overrepresented in the psychiatric treatment population, especially in recent years.[2-5,13-14]

Comorbidity rates are also quite discrepant between clinical and nonclinical samples. The most extensive population based study of comorbidity is the Epidemiologic Catchment Area Study (ECA). The ECA Study rates for the combined psychiatric and addictive disorders are indicated in Table 2, Columns 2 and 3. For comparative purposes, the prevalence rates derived from clinical psychiatric settings seen in Table 1 are included here as Column 1. A comparison of the ratios for prevalence rates of comorbidity in psychiatric settings compared to the general population clearly reveals the bias

TABLE 2: PREVALENCE RATES FOR COMORBIDITY IN THE PSYCHIATRIC SETTING COMPARED TO THE GENERAL POPULATION (ECA STUDY)

DIAGNOSIS: COMORBIDITY	PREVALENCE RATE: CLINICAL SETTING[a]	PREVALENCE RATE: NONCLINICAL-MALE[b]	PREVALENCE RATE: NONCLINICAL-FEMALE[c]	RATIO: CLINICAL TO NONCLINICAL[d]
Depressive Disorders	30%	8%	23.4%	3.8/1.3
Bipolar Disorders	50	0.8	3.1	62.5/16.1
Schizophrenia	50	2.4	7.2	20.8/6.9
Antisocial Personality	80	14.6	10.1	5.5/7.9
Anxiety Disorders	30	2.1*	7.9*	14.3/3.8
Phobic Disorders	23	13.5	33.1	1.7/.7

a: per cent of patients diagnosed with comorbid addictive disorder

b: per cent of male population with comorbid psychiatric and addictive disorder

c: per cent of female population with comorbid psychiatric and addictive disorder

d: ratio of clinical to nonclinical male/ratio of clinical to nonclinical female

*panic disorder

towards high rates in clinical settings for certain psychiatric diagnoses. For example, the ratio for comorbidity for males with schizophrenia illustrates how a psychiatric clinician would falsely conclude that addictive comorbidity is quite common. Instead, these data appear to confirm the hypothesis that dually diagnosed patients are very much overrepresented in the treatment population than are nonaddicted patients with schizophrenia.[7,15]

METHODOLOGY OF STUDY DESIGN

The basic design of data acquisition is also important in understanding comorbidity rates. Retrospective analysis yields higher rates for psychiatric comorbidity than a prospective analysis where the stability of diagnoses can be tested over time. This is because (1) alcohol and drugs can produce psychiatric syndromes (2) patient self reports tend to de-emphasize substance use in the genesis of psychiatric symptoms, and, (3) patients and clinicians alike tend to view psychiatric symptoms as either independent or the cause of substance use. In contrast longitudinal studies reveal that psychiatric syndromes are more likely to be a result of substance use.[1,16]

The importance of prospective design is illustrated by the much lower prevalence rates for comorbidity in addicted patients when a period of withdrawal and abstinence is allowed before psychiatric diagnosis is made. The recommended period before establishing independent psychiatric comorbidity distinct from that arising secondary to the pharmacological effects and other acquired addiction induced changes is between four weeks to two years. However, the drop off in diagnoseable psychiatric illness over time depends on the diagnosis. Depressive and psychotic symptoms tend to resolve in days to weeks whereas anxiety symptoms and personality changes diminish over months to years.

Depressive symptoms occur in 98% of alcoholics at some time. One third will meet criteria for persistent depression which interferes with functioning for at least two weeks; for the vast majority, the depressive symptoms resolve with abstinence and alcoholism treatment. Administration of moderate doses (three to five drinks) of alcohol can produce depressive symptoms in normal subjects under experimental conditions. Similar alcohol doses given to healthy women may produce mood disruptions that can still be measured days after the conclusion of the experiment. These and other studies show that continuous, heavy drinking produces a "depressive syndrome" of alcohol intoxication. This "depressive syndrome" is associated with other drugs such as stimulants, cannabis, sedative/hypnotics and opiates.[1,16]

The cross sectional analysis typically done for addictive disorders in psychiatric populations without longitudinal follow-up results in unstable and inflated rates of psychiatric comorbidity that is in fact related to, rather than truly co-morbid with the addictive disorders. Even longitudinal studies will inflate rates of anxiety and personality disorders relative to psychotic and affective disorders if insufficient time is allowed. The most skilled clinician cannot make accurate and reliable diagnoses that have predictive value using a point prevalence method of analysis; large epidemiologic studies rarely employ such skilled clinicians. A cross sectional epidemiologic study is best viewed as instructive of the high rate of psychiatric symptomatology and organic psychiatric disorders associated with addictive disorders without regard to etiology and therefore actual comorbidity.

Retrospective recall derived from addicted patients will also falsely inflate rates of psychiatric comorbidity. For example, abstinent alcoholics will retrospectively attribute drinking to anxiety and depression but be found to be free of these symptoms on examination. When these same alcoholics are given alcohol under experimental conditions, anxiety and depression develop in proportion to the increase in the amount and duration of alcohol consumption. Upon detoxification, the psychiatric symptoms resolve. The subjects do not recall the severe symptoms which developed during intoxication and will continue to explain drinking on the basis of anxiety and depression. The attribution of drinking and drug use to psychiatric symptoms extends to hallucinations and delusions in psychotic patients, and personality difficulties in patients with personality disorders.[17]

If data are gathered retrospectively shortly after a recent episode of substance use, the self report will result in exaggerated rates of psychiatric disorders due to the addict's rationalization of the use. While it may be accurate to assume that an alcoholic or drug addict interviewed in an addiction treatment setting will reliably acknowledge frequency and duration of use, the individual's interpretation of why she or he uses remains distorted until sober for a prolonged period of time, often until the addict understands her or his addictive use of alcohol and drugs through treatment or self-help involvement.[17-18]

Prospective analyses reveal that psychological states and personality variables do not predict the onset of drinking or alcoholism. These studies do not find that psychiatric diagnoses or symptoms precede or lead to higher rates of addiction. When longitudinal follow-up occurs over time after onset through the abstinent, treated state, the psychiatric symptoms and personality abnormalities associated with addictive use and intoxication resolve in most of those affected, with the young chronically mentally ill as exceptions. However, it is worth noting that addictive comorbidity in the young chronically mentally ill patient affects symptoms most commonly associated with the addictive illness: hostility, noncompliance, disruptive behaviors. Where studied, young chronically mentally ill patients with addictive comorbidity cannot be distinguished from their nonaddicted mentally ill peers by primary psychiatric diagnosis or by symptoms such as hallucinations, delusions, or paranoia.[3,13,19]

BIASES OF THE INVESTIGATOR

The perspective of the clinician or researcher is a key determinant in the assessment of comorbidity prevalence rates. If one's perspective is that addiction is an independent disorder which directly causes psychiatric symptoms and syndromes, one uses exclusionary criteria before making independent psychiatric diagnoses. As a result of excluding psychopathology that arises from the addictive disorder, the prevalence rates for psychiatric disorders in those patients with addictive disorders are generally in the range for those rates in the general population.

If one's perspective is that psychiatric disorders or symptoms directly cause addiction, one finds high prevalence rates for psychiatric disorders in addiction populations because exclusionary criteria (found in DSM-III-R) are not applied. The "self-medication" hypothesis–that is, that substances are used to self-medicate underlying and primary mental illness–remains a pervasive perspective that falsely elevates the prevalence rate of psychiatric diagnosis in addiction populations. While self-medication of an underlying condition (most often a psychiatric rather than medical condition) is often cited in the literature as an explanation of substance use, when tested, the hypothesis cannot be validated. In fact, several studies show that addicts and alcoholics use despite worsening or drug and alcohol induced psychiatric symptoms.[20]

LENGTH OF FOLLOW UP

Follow-up provides perhaps the only valid way to establish the stability of comorbidity prevalence rates. If mental and addictive disorders are truly comorbid, either will persist after the other is in remission. By design, a post-intoxication period is not employed in cross sectional or retrospective studies, which therefore will elevate prevalence rates for psychiatric syndromes induced by drugs and alcohol. The lack of a careful, prospective follow-up in clinical studies is also in part responsible for the artifactually high rates of psychiatric comorbidity found among those with an addictive diagnosis and vice versa.[1,21]

It has been demonstrated that subjects who are psychiatrically symptom free develop clearly definable psychiatric syndromes indistinguishable from those defined in DSM-III-R when exposed to alcohol and drugs. Cocaine infusions in human volunteers induce paranoid delusions as a pharmacological effect of cocaine, that closely follow the blood levels of cocaine. Other studies with alcohol demonstrate that severe depression develops with intoxication in otherwise symptom free subjects. These affective changes have been correlated with blood alcohol levels, and correspond to known pharmacokinetics of alcohol.[1,16]

Moreover, when clinical populations are examined over time, psychiatric symptoms such as anxiety and depression correspond to periods of alcohol intoxication, diminish with periods of abstinence, and reappear with relapse. In general, similar results are found for the courses in other drug dependencies where the psychiatric syndromes follow the course of drug use, and are not etiological or independent in themselves.[21-22]

The question of the length of follow-up has been examined for many drugs including alcohol for the major psychiatric syndromes. For alcohol, 2 to 4 weeks may be needed for the pharmacological effects to recede, although a normal mood may appear within days. A similar course for resolution of cocaine induced psychiatric symptoms has been documented. For longer acting drugs such as benzodiazepines or methadone the course may be protracted.[1,16,23]

TREATMENT INTERVENTIONS

A differential response to treatment interventions can distinguish the comorbidity of psychiatric disorders from addictive disorders. Studies performed on alcoholics employing pharmacological treatments for psychiatric illness do not show a favorable response in either the psychiatric symptoms or addictive course. Preliminary studies in cocaine addicts suggest certain therapeutic pharmacological agents (desipramine for cocaine, and clonidine for heroin) have a beneficial effect in promoting abstinence in acute and subacute withdrawal in cocaine and heroin addicts, similar to the use of benzodiazepines in alcoholics. However, these therapeutic agents do not have demonstrated efficacy in prophylaxis or relapse prevention from these addictive drugs, as would be predicted if "underlying" psychiatric disorders caused the drinking or drug use.[24]

Treatment outcome studies indicate that specific treatment of the alcohol and/or drug addiction will result in the amelioration of the associated psychiatric syndromes and alter the course of the addictive disorder. Abstinence and specific treatment of the addictive disorder resulted in the resolution or diminution of affective, anxiety, psychotic and personality disturbances in the vast majority of the patients.[25]

Some studies assume that treatment of the psychiatric symptoms will result in a lowered morbidity and mortality from the addictive disorder. This view holds that the addictive disorders are dependent on the psychiatric disorders, and etiologically linked to them. There is, however, little systematic evidence beyond the anecdotal to support this popular but unproven position. Our concern is that to insist on the priority of the psychiatric disorder in diagnosis and treatment will prevent the definitive treatment which will reduce the psychiatric morbidity and mortality caused by addictive disorders.[15]

Finally, it is clinically established that the successful treatment of true, independent psychiatric disorders is only possible once the addictive disorder is under control (i.e., abstinence from hallucinogens and depressants). Moreover, compliance with psychiatric treatments is usually poor in the setting of active addictive disorders. Studies show that those chronic psychiatric patients with untreated addictive disorders experience a greater number of relapses, greater severity of illness, poor medication use, heavier utilization of psychiatric services and generally poorer outcome than those without an addictive disorder.[26-28]

REFERENCES

1. Miller NS, Mahler JC, Belkin BM, et al. Psychiatric diagnosis in alcohol & drug dependence. Ann Clin Psychiatry 1990;3:79-89.

2. Drake RE, Wallach MA. Substance abuse among the chronic mentally ill. Hosp Community Psychiatry 1989;40:1041-1046.

3. Pepper B, Kirshner MC, Ryglewicz H. The young adult chronic patient: overview of a population. Hosp Community Psychiatry 1981;32:7;463-474.

4. Drake RE, Osher EC, Wallach MA. Alcohol use and abuse in schizophrenia: a prospective community study. J Nerv Ment Dis. 1989;177:7;408-414.

5. Barbee JG, Clark PD, Crapanzano BS, et al. Alcohol and substance abuse among schizophrenic patients presenting to an emergency psychiatric service. J Nerv Ment Dis. 1989;177:7;400-407.

6. Myers JK, Weissman MM, Tschler GL, et al. Six-month prevalence of psychiatric disorders in three communities. Arch Gen Psychiatry 1984;41:959-967.

7. Robins LN, Helzer JE, Przybeck TR, et al. Alcohol disorders in the community: a report from the epidemiologic catchment area. In Rose RM, Barrett J. eds. Alcoholism: origins and outcome. New York: Raven Press Ltd, 1988.

8. Caton CL, Gralnick A, Bender S, et al. Young chronic patients and substance abuse. Hosp Community Psychiatry 1989;40:10;1037-1040.

9. Alterman AI, Erdlen FR, Murphy E. Alcohol abuse in the psychiatric hospital population. Addict Behav. 1981;6:69-73.

10. Lamb HR. Young adult chronic patients: the new drifters. Hosp Community Psychiatry 1982;33:6;465-468.

11. Schwartz SR, Goldfinger SM. The new chronic patient: clinical characteristics of an emergency subgroup. Hosp Community Psychiatry 1981;470-474.

12. Sheets JL, Prevost JA, Reihman J. Young adult chronic patients: three hypothesized subgroups. Hosp Community Psychiatry 1982;33:3;197-203.

13. Hekimian LJ, Gershon S. Characteristics of drug abusers admitted to a psychiatric hospital. JAMA. 1968;205:75-80.

14. Rosenheck R, Massari L, Astrachan B, et al. Mentally ill chemical abusers discharged from VA inpatient treatment: 1976-88. Psychiatr Q. 1990;61: 4; 237- 249.

15. Regier DA, Farmer ME, Rae DS, et al. Cormorbidity of mental disorders with alcohol and other drug abuse: results from the epidemiological catchment area (ECA) study. JAMA. 1991;264:19;2511-2518.

16. Schuckit MA, Montero MG. Alcoholism, anxiety, depression. Br J Addict. 1980;83:1373-1380.

17. Tamerin JS, Mendelson JH. The psychodynamics of chronic inebriation. Observations of alcoholics during the process of drinking in an experimental group setting. Am J Psychiatry. 1969;125:886.

18. Vaillant GE, Milofsky E. The etiology of alcoholism. Am Psychol. 1982;37:5;494-503.

19. McCarrick AK, Manderscheid RW, Bertolucci DE. Correlates of acting-out behaviors among young adult chronic patients. Hosp Community Psychiatry. 1985;36:8;848-853.

20. Khantzian EJ. The self-medication hypothesis of addiction disorders: focus on heroin and cocaine dependence. Am J Psychiatry. 1985;142:1259-1264.

21. Schuckit MA. Alcoholism and sociopathy-diagnostic confusion. Q J Stud Alcohol. 1973;34:157-164.

22. Brown SA, Irwin M, Schuckit MA. Changes in anxiety among abstinent male alcoholics. J Stud Alcohol. 1991;52:1;55-61.

23. Schuckit MA, Irwin M, Brown SA. The history of anxiety symptoms among 171 primary alcoholics. J Stud Alcohol. 1990;31:1;34-41.

24. Miller NS. The pharmacology of alcohol and drugs of abuse and addiction. New York: Springer-Verlag, 1991.

25. Harrison PA, Hoffman NG, Streed SG. Drug and alcohol addiction treatment outcome. In Miller NS, ed. Comprehensive handbook of drug and alcohol addiction. New York: Marcel-Dekker, Inc, 1991.

26. Minkoff K. An integrated treatment model for dual diagnosis of psychosis and addiction. Hosp Community Psychiatry. 1989;40:10;1031-1036.

27. Kosten TR, Kleber HD. Differential diagnosis of psychiatric comorbidity in substance abusers. J Subst Abuse Treat. 1988;5:201-206.

28. Helzer JE, Pryzbeck TR. The co-occurrence of alcoholism with other psychiatric disorders in the general population and its impact on treatment. J Stud Alcohol. 49:3;219-224.

Evaluation and Acute Management of Psychotic Symptomatology in Alcohol and Drug Addictions

James Fine, MD
Norman S. Miller, MD

SUMMARY. The practical clinical evaluation of patients manifesting psychotic symptomatology and addictive illness is approached in diverse and contradictory ways. While addiction specialists may not recognize the existence of Axis I disorders that prevent the utilization of treatment in the system, trained mental health professionals are traditionally prone to deny or minimize the addictive process and its capacity to produce psychiatric symptoms. This may result in premature diagnosis, and in a poor response to psychiatric treatment.

The purpose of this paper is to describe a pragmatic model, based on clinically observable conditions, for the evaluation and acute

---

James Fine is Director, Kings County Addictive Disease Hospital, Department of Psychiatry, Downstate Medical Center, State University of New York, Brooklyn, NY.

Norman S. Miller is Director, Section for Alcohol/Drug Programs, Department of Psychiatry, University of Illinois at Chicago, West Side VA Medical Center, Chicago, IL.

Reprint requests should be addressed to James Fine, Kings County Addictive Disease Hospital, Downstate Medical Center, 450 Clarkson Avenue, K-Building, Box 9, Brooklyn, NY 11203.

[Haworth co-indexing entry note]: "Evaluation and Acute Management of Psychotic Symptomatology in Alcohol and Drug Addictions." Fine, James, and Norman S. Miller.. Co-published simultaneously in *Journal of Addictive Diseases,* (The Haworth Press, Inc.) Vol. 12, No. 3, 1993, pp. 59-71; and: *Comorbidity of Addictive and Psychiatric Disorders* (Ed: Norman S. Miller, and Barry Stimmel) The Haworth Press, Inc., 1993, pp. 59-71. Multiple copies of this article/chapter may be purchased from The Haworth Document Delivery Center. Call 1-800-3- HAWORTH (1-800-342-9678) between 9:00 - 5:00(EST) and ask for DOCUMENT DELIVERY CENTER.

59

management of major psychiatric symptomatology associated with diagnosed drug and alcohol addiction. Before describing the model, psychotic illness and symptoms in the general population versus the drug and alcohol addicted will be examined. The model will be applied to a few discrete syndromes based on common clinical presentations.

RELATIONSHIP BETWEEN DRUG AND ALCOHOL USE AND PSYCHIATRIC DISTURBANCE

Psychiatric disturbance is frequently associated with psychoactive drug and alcohol use.[1,2] The association even appears in popular terminology, such as the reference by Alcoholics Anonymous to "the insanity of alcoholism," and the term "dope fiend" which evokes images of derangement and perversity. Current estimates of the prevalence of coexisting diagnoses of mental and substance abuse disorders range from 12% to 61%.[3,4] Differential diagnosis has been stressed as requisite for the effective pharmacological and therapeutic treatment of the dually diagnosed.[5]

Patients with significant patterns of drug and alcohol use can present with a variety of symptoms and psychopathology usually indicative of either and Axis I or Axis II disorder in DSM-III-R or both. In this paper, clinical observation and currently existing data are used to provide the basis for evaluation and treatment of coexisting psychotic symptomatology. The focus is on acute management of major psychiatric symptoms typically associated with Axis I disorders. Although chemical dependency may coexist with additional psychiatric disorders such as anxiety disorders, somatoform disorders, dissociative disorders, attention deficit disorders, and bipolar disorders, they will not be addressed at the present time. Similarly, the diagnosis and management of character disorders is a somewhat separate topic for a further paper.

PSYCHOTIC ILLNESS AND SYMPTOMS IN THE GENERAL POPULATION VERSUS THE DRUG AND ALCOHOL ADDICTED

Estimates of the incidences of acute and chronic psychotic illness in the general population vary considerably. If Organic Mental Syndromes and Psychoactive Substance Use Disorders are excluded, psychotic symptoms are generally attributable to Schizophrenia, Delusional Disorders, Mood Disorders, and Psychotic Disorders Not Elsewhere Classified. The overall prevalence of these disorders is not generally believed to be high and can be assumed for the purpose of this analysis to be approximately 5%.

This figure of 5% is somewhat arbitrary but statistically defensible. Specifically, we appeal to Reiger et al. where data are presented for the combined Community and Institutionalized Population. (Since we are looking at incidence of symptomatology, the one month prevalence category seems most relevant since it is furthest from long term prevalence.) If we sum "Schizophrenic/Schizophreniform Disorders" (0.7%) and "Affective Disorders" (5.2%) and subtract from the latter "Dysthymia" (3.8%), we arrive at a total of 3.6%. Allowing another percentage point for "Delusional Disorders" and "Psychotic Disorders Not Elsewhere Classified" (which are not featured in the table), we come quite close to the 5% hypothetical figure. (Note, however, that doubling or halving it will not significantly change the conclusions that follow). The number of actively addicted dependent individuals in the general population is also assumed to be 5%. (Again, some might argue for a somewhat higher figure (10%); this would not significantly alter the discussion).

If we examine the chemically addicted population, we can assume a higher prevalence of the major psychiatric illnesses specified above.[6] How much higher, however, is a subject of clinical and academic speculation. For the purpose of this analysis, a rate of psychiatric illness of twice "typical" (i.e., twice that of the general population) will be assumed for the drug and alcohol addicted population. (Again, assuming a higher rate–i.e., three times normal–will not significantly change the model being presented.)

These assumed prevalences lead to the following conclusions. Approximately one out of 20 individuals in the general population (non-chemically dependent) being evaluated for active psychotic illness will be found to have such illness. Thus, in a group of 20 actively chemically dependent individuals, two individuals will suffer from such psychotic illness. Conversely, 19 out of 20 individuals in the general population would be free of active psychotic illness, while 18 out of 20 chemically dependent individuals would be free of psychotic illness. A more extreme assumption (e.g., three times the prevalence of psychotic illness in the chemically dependent) would result in 17 out of 20 individuals being free of psychotic illness.

From the perspective of clinical service, it is important whether one, two, or three people out of 20 (i.e., 5, 10 or 15%) will require treatment for major psychotic illness. It is vital to determine as specifically as possible these numbers and to plan the health needs of various populations. (A two or three fold increase in need for psychiatric hospital beds for a specific population is obviously significant.) However, from the perspective of acute management and diagnosis, the significant fact is that psychotic illness is *not* found in most (70-95%) of the general population of the chemically dependent population.

What confounds this situation, however, is the mode of distribution of psychotic symptoms among these population. Figure 1 visually represents the comparative prevalence of psychotic illness in both populations. Little data is available to provide numbers on the prevalence of specific psychotic symptoms such as hallucinations, delusions, incoherence, thought disorder, mania, and profound depression (with anhedonia, anergia and suicidality). However, it can be assumed that such symptoms are relatively uncommon in the general population (i.e., they would be found in a minority of individuals). General clinical consensus would likely support this assumption.

FIGURE 1.   Comparative Prevalence of Psychotic Illness in General and Chemically Dependent Populations

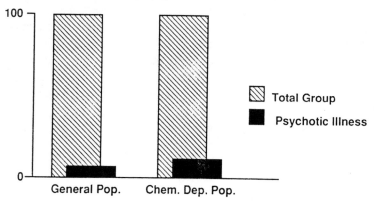

Individuals with active chemical dependency (often with intermittent and prolonged periods of intoxication and withdrawal), however, frequently manifest psychotic symptoms periodically. Symptoms of addiction often mimic psychotic ones.[7,8] Often patients themselves cannot distinguish between panic and withdrawal symptoms.[9] Hallucinations, paranoid delusions, disturbances in the form of thought, and profound alterations in mood are common occurrences in the course of addictive illness, as regarded longitudinally. Figure 2 reflects the plethoric nature of psychotic symptoms in the chemically dependent population when compared to the general. Thus, while psychotic illness is likely to be modestly, or even moderately, increased in the chemically dependent, psychotic symptoms are dramatically increased. Therefore, psychotic symptoms have *less diagnostic validity for mental illness in the chemically dependent population* than they do in the general population.

BASIC PRINCIPLES
FOR EVALUATING PSYCHOTIC SYMPTOMS
IN THE DRUG AND ALCOHOL ADDICTED

An analysis of the preceding discussion suggests a simple and

FIGURE 2. Ratios of Psychotic Illness to Psychotic Symptoms in General and
Chemically Dependent Populations

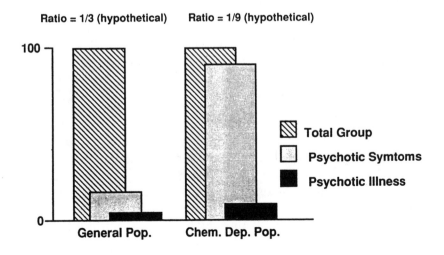

direct strategy for evaluating the chemically dependent individual with psychotic symptoms. The first principle is that due to the poor diagnostic validity of such symptoms, it is necessary for the clinician to entertain a relatively high index of suspicion of psychotic illness. Current symptomatology cannot be relied upon either to assume the presence of, or to specify, a psychiatric diagnosis, and the majority of symptoms observed will not be indicative of major psychiatric illness. One cannot deduce the existence of a preexisting psychiatric illness based on presenting psychotic symptoms. During acute episodes in the chemically dependent, a definitive psychiatric diagnosis is simply not possible. It is made *only* if symptoms recur or persist after *significant* abstinence.

While most psychotic symptoms in the chemically dependent population may be transient, there is little evidence that these symptoms, while present, are less dangerous than those produced by psychotic illness. In fact, violence in response to hallucinations and delusions, and suicidality in response to chemically induced depressive symptoms, are well documented.[10] This leads to the second basic principle: one must provide acute treatment of psychotic symptoms. Clinicians need to keep in mind that the existence of chemical dependency does not reduce the dangerousness of psychotic symptoms.

After initial stabilization, the clinician will be expected to plan the long-term treatment and to arrive at a diagnosis. The addictive illness and/or psychiatric disorder need to be treated (or referred for treatment).

A MODEL FOR THE ACUTE MANAGEMENT AND TREATMENT OF MAJOR PSYCHIATRIC SYMPTOMATOLOGY IN ALCOHOL AND DRUG ADDICTIONS

The overall goal of the proposed model is to help chemically dependent individuals become free of psychoactive chemical use and its attendant psychological disruption. While conceptually simple and rational, the practical application of this methodology is complicated by the fact that psychotic symptoms secondary to chemical dependency and abuse may persist for prolonged periods of time; in addition, many (if not most) patients with chemical dependency are not likely to become chemical-free easily, rapidly, or for long periods. Consequently, the goal of this treatment model may be achieved only in relative terms and for a portion of patients. The approach, however, still represents the appropriate management of this patient population. Simply stated, chemically dependent individuals, with or without coexisting psychiatric illness, do not improve unless they achieve or approach abstinence. Addicted patients with psychotic symptoms who remain active in their psychoactive chemical use, are unlikely to benefit from psychiatric medications, social intervention or counseling (whether or not they also have psychotic illnesses).

The suggested treatment approach is outlined below:

1. Treat life threatening complications.
   (a) Treat overdose and withdrawal.
   (b) Hospitalize psychiatrically for suicidality or dangerousness (on a locked ward with appropriately trained staff).
2. Support abstinence.
   (a) Refer to treatment programs.
   (b) Refer to AA/NA/CA and Double Trouble Groups.
   (c) Provide ongoing personal support.
3. Use appropriate psychiatric medications if symptoms persist and impair function and recovery.
4. Do not use cross-tolerant sedatives except for detoxification.
5. Discontinue medications and observe patient for recurrence of psychiatric symptoms.
6. Formulate psychiatric diagnoses based on reappearance or persistence of symptoms in absence of active chemical use.
7. Provide appropriate psychiatric medications and management based on clinical course over time.

PRESENTING SYNDROMES AND PRACTICAL APPLICATIONS OF THE MODEL

While psychiatric symptoms are plethoric and chemical dependency coexists with virtually all psychiatric disorders, we are limiting the discussion to three general syndromes: Depressive, Paranoid and Anxious. It is the clinical impression of the authors that most acute presentations can be adequately subsumed under these categories, although certainly many more actual diagnoses would be embedded within these clinical syndromes (i.e., somatoform, dissociative disorders, etc.). The coexistence of intoxications, withdrawal and persistent cognitive dysfunction must always be assessed, often constitute medical emergencies, and must first be treated and controlled. (Their management is not dealt with here.)

The *Depressive Syndrome* seen in chemical use is identical to the depressive syndrome produced by Affective Illness. It is characterized by sad mood, guilt, hopelessness, worthlessness, agitation or psychomotor retardation, anhedonia, sleep disturbance (increased or decreased), delusions, and suicidality. It may be associated with all forms of chemical dependency and abuse, but is frequently associated with chronic sedative use, chronic stimulant use, or intoxication and withdrawal.

The *Paranoid Syndrome* is also clinically indistinguishable from that produced by "pure" psychiatric illness. It is characterized by suspiciousness, delusions, hallucinations, clear sensorium, and hypervigilance. Hypervigilance can be conceived of as the affective and emotional tone of an agitated paranoid state *without* psychotic process. It is characterized by irritability, suspiciousness and hyperarousal. These paranoid types of presentation may also be associated with all forms of chemical dependency and abuse. They are frequently associated with chronic stimulant use, hallucinagen use, intoxication and withdrawal.

The *Anxious Syndrome* consists of the symptoms seen in functional anxiety disorders. It can be characterized by symptoms of panic (including shortness of breath, dizziness, palpitations, trembling, etc.), unrealistic and overwhelming anxiety, edginess and inability to concentrate, or obsessive symptoms.

While mixed pictures frequently present, these three syndromes can serve as useful models into which most presentations can be categorized for practical evaluation. Let us now apply the proposed methodology to alcohol and drug involved patients being seen in a mental health or addiction clinic, presenting with a new onset of one of the previously described syndromes.

1. Treat Life Threatening Complications

Is the patient suicidally depressed, combative due to hallucinations or delusions, or dangerously impulsive due to anxiety? Is he/she so depressed, anxious or disorganized to the point of being unable to feed, clothe or care of him/herself? If so, hospitalization is required (or, at least, a supervised setting in the last instance). These criteria are standard psychiatric evaluation criteria. The one significant difference in evaluating the acute chemically involved population is the use, when available, of a safe holding area since symptoms may remit rapidly.

2. Support Abstinence

Once the decision whether or not to hospitalize is made, the next step is supportive CONFRONTATION. This involves contrasting the adverse consequences of use (life problems, symptoms) with the *alternative* of avoiding these consequences through a program leading to abstinence.

A treatment plan should be developed to help achieve abstinence, including referral to treatment programs, safe residential arrangements, and AA and/or NA and/or "Double Trouble" groups specifically designed to meet the needs of psychiatrically disturbed chemically dependent individuals. Clinicians may assume that psychiatrically impaired patients cannot tolerate, or be tolerated by, self help groups, and they may believe that the Twelve Step Fellowships are confrontative and intrusive which is not necessarily the case. Dual diagnosis patients can often participate in and benefit from AA and NA if they are given special preparation,[11] and they have a better chance of maintaining sobriety if they learn to use AA.[12] Such preparation can be done individually or in groups and should include role-playing as well as clear statements to the patients about what they may expect at meetings.

Patients who deny dependency and report that they can stop "on their own," should be supportively encouraged to attempt to do so, while being carefully monitored. If unable to stop, they are then confronted with the failure of their plan and the necessity of treatment.

While supporting abstinence can be described quickly, it is often a long and difficult process. Denial and minimization, as well as frank psychotic symptoms, can often block acceptance of the need for treatment. It is clinically vital, however, to keep in mind that providing medications and financial benefits in the *absence* of education and confrontation, can give the message that chemical dependency is "secondary." This constitutes *enabling,* which can be described as supporting denial and deflecting attention. Once the support of abstinence *(not necessarily its attainment)* is established, the methodology should be continued.

3. Use Appropriate Psychiatric Medications if Symptoms Persist and Impair Function and Recovery

Patients may experience symptoms that prevent their engagement in necessary life activities, including chemical dependency treatment. An inpatient, who after several days in a detoxification unit, gets more depressed and begins to exhibit significant vegetative symptoms due to profound depression, should be evaluated carefully for antidepressant therapy. If supportive counseling and nutrition do not rapidly improve the clinical picture, medications should be started. A diagnosis of *affective episode* (e.g., Organic Affective Disorder) should be made, since there would be no reason to assume at that point in time that the patient has an *affective illness.*

Similarly, a patient suffering from the Paranoid Syndrome might be delusionally suspicious and fearful, or simply distracted by an hallucinosis and unable to attend a community or AA meeting. If these symptoms do not improve within a few days, or if they grow worse, the patient should receive antipsychotic medications to permit safe, effective, and comfortable functioning. An *episode* of psychosis should be diagnosed (e.g., Organic Hallucinosis, Organic Delusional Disorder), and not an ongoing psychotic *illness.*

Anxiety symptoms in chemically dependent individuals are prevalent and usually self limited. However, Anxiety Disorders are common and often treatable.[13] Anxiety, when disabling as in the examples above, should be managed with behavioral therapy, beta blockers, tricyclic antidepressants, and seratonergic drugs such as buspirone and fluoxetine. Emergency sedation may be necessary for extreme agitation. Again, the diagnosis of a temporary disturbance (i.e., Organic Anxiety Disorder) should be made.

The identical criteria (the inability to engage in necessary activities, especially recovery-oriented ones) apply when evaluating outpatients. In clinic settings as well, initial diagnoses should be of *temporary* conditions, with issues of "primacy" best deferred,[14,15,16] in favor of engaging the patient into treatment as soon as possible.

4. Do Not Use Cross Tolerant Medication Except for Detoxification

Except for acute detoxification or *emergency* sedation, the use of cross tolerant sedatives (e.g., benzodiazepines, meprobamate, barbiturates, etc.) should be avoided in both outpatient and inpatient settings. Sleep disturbance should be managed behaviorally, or with bedtime doses of sedating antidepressants if the disturbance is profound.

Various issues in medicating the addictive patient have been raised in the psychiatric literature.[18] The use of sedatives is contraindicated for practical clinical reasons. Chemically dependent individuals develop rapid and extreme tolerance to these medications, thus becoming refractory to the therapeutic effects while experiencing an exacerbation of anxiety (and insomnia) due to withdrawal phenomena. This reduction in efficacy and increase in symptoms often lead to increased dosage, possible addiction to these drugs, and more likelihood of relapse to their drug of choice.

5. Discontinue Medications and Observe Patient for Recurrence of Psychiatric Symptoms

Assuming major psychiatric symptoms have ceased, or, at least, have very significantly reduced for a period of months, medications should be discontinued and the patient observed over time. This approach coincides with the appropriate response to individuals with other psychiatric disorders (e.g., Major Depression, Panic Disorder, etc.).

6. Formulate Psychiatric Diagnoses Based on Reappearance of Symptoms in the Absence of Chemical Use

If symptoms recur, and the patient is verifiably abstinent, a definitive non-organic psychiatric disorder can be diagnosed. For example, if three months after trycyclics are discontinued, an abstinent patient becomes clinically depressed and meets DSM-III-R criteria, a Major Depressive Episode can be diagnosed. The recurrence of significant anxiety symptoms would support the diagnosis of an Anxiety Disorder. Similarly, the reappearance of delusions in such a patient would warrant a diagnosis of a Delusional Disorder. If hallucinations were also present, Schizophrenia (or Schizophreniform Psychosis) would be diagnosed. If, however, as is often the case, abstinence has not be reliably demonstrated, the methodology should be reapplied (or rather, should continue to be applied) with no new or definitive diagnosis. Continued support of abstinence and recovery, coupled with appropriate periods of medication use, will reduce hospitalization and improve functioning even in the absence of achieving abstinence or arriving at a "final" diagnosis.

7. Provide Appropriate Psychiatric Medications and Management Based on Clinical Course Over Time

When definitive psychiatric diagnoses independent of chemical dependence are made, patients should receive the standard accepted psychiatric treatment in addition to treatment for chemical dependency. Clinical inference dictates that receiving both treatments in a unified program works best. Studies are underway to test this hypothesis (Rosenthal, note 1). If such programs are unavailable, tandem or parallel treatments should occur, since neither psychiatric care nor addiction treatment will be successful unless *both* are successful. Appropriate liaisons and mechanisms for the exchange of clinical information must be developed. Patients should be educated as to their need to take medications and how this differs from abuse and dependence. Addiction counselors also need to understand the importance of medications, while psychiatrically oriented therapists must recognize the significance of active addictive use and relapse, and how these block effective psychiatric treatment.

NOTE

1. Rosenthal, R. (191). Unified treatment program studies for dual diagnostic patients. Department of Psychiatry, Beth Israel Hospital, personal communication.

REFERENCES

1. Bunt G, Galanter M, Lifshutz H, Castanedo, R. Cocaine/Crack dependence among psychiatric inpatients. Am J Psychiatry, 1990;147 (11):1542-1546.

2. Reiger DA, Farmer ME, Rae DS, Locke BZ, Keith SJ, Judd LL, Goodwin FK. Comorbidity of mental disorders with alcohol and other drug abuse: Results from the epidemiologic catchment area (ECA) study. JAMA, 1990;264(19):2511-2518, 2513.

3. Keisler CA, Simpkins CG, Morton TL. Prevalence of dual diagnoses of mental and substance abuse disorders in general hospitals. Hosp Community Psychiatry, 1991;42(4):400-403.

4. Crowne DB, Rosse RB, Sheridan MJ, Deutsch SI. Substance abuse diagnoses and discharge patterns among psychiatric inpatients. Hosp Community Psychiatry, 1991;42(4):403-405.

5. Kosten TR, Kleber HD. Differential diagnosis of psychiatric comorbidity in substance abusers. J Subst Abuse Treat. 1988;5(4):201-206.

6. Nace EP. Substance use disorders and personality disorders: Comorbidity. Psychiatry Hosp. 1989;20(2):65-69.

7. Miller NS, Mahler JC, Belkin BM, Gold MS. Psychiatric diagnosis in alcohol and drug dependence. Annals of Clinical Psychiatry, 1991;3:79-89.

8. Miller NS, Ries RK. Drug and alcohol dependence and psychiatric populations: The need for diagnosis, intervention, and training. Comp Psychiatry, 1991;32(3):268-276.

9. George DT, ZerbyA, Noble S, Nutt DJ. Panic attacks and alcohol withdrawal: Can subjects differentiate the symptoms? Biol Psychiatry, 1988;24(2):240-243.

10. Brody SL. Violence associated with acute cocaine use in patients admitted to a medical emergency department. NIDA Research Monograph Series, 1990;103:44-59.

11. Minkoff K. An integrated treatment model for dual diagnosis of psychosis and addiction.Hosp Community Psychiatry, 1989;40(10):1031-1036.

12. Kofoed L, Kania J, Walsh T, et al. Outpatient treatment of patients with substance abuse and coexisting psychiatric disorders. AM J Psychiatry, 1986; 143:867-872.

13. Weser RB. Alcohol use and abuse secondary to anxiety. Psychiatry Clin North Am. 1990;13(4):699-713.

14. Lehman AI, Myers EP, Corty E. Assessment and classification of patients with psychiatric and substance abuse syndromes. Hosp Community Psychiatry, 1989;40(10):1019-1025.

15. Shuckit MA, Montiero MG. Alcoholism, anxiety, and depression. Br J Addict. 1988;83:1373-1380.

16. Weiss RD, Mirin SM. The dual diagnosis alcoholic and treatment. Psychiatric Annals, 1989;19(5):261-265.

17. Hanson M, Kramer TH, Gross W. Outpatient treatment of adults with coexisting substance use and mental disorders. J Subst Abuse Treat. 1990;7;190-116.

18. Zweben JE, Smith DE. Considerations in using psychotropic medication with dual diagnosis patients in recovery. J Psychoactive Drugs,1989;21(2):221-228.

Affective and Anxiety Disorders and Alcohol and Drug Dependence: Diagnosis and Treatment

Robert M. Anthenelli, MD
Marc A. Schuckit, MD

SUMMARY. Depression and anxiety frequently coexist in patients with substance use disorders. This clinically-oriented article examines the relationship between these conditions and emphasizes data showing that substances of abuse can cause signs and symptoms of both depression and anxiety. These substance-related syndromes appear

Robert M. Anthenelli is a Research Fellow, Department of Psychiatry, San Diego Veterans Affairs Medical Center and University of California, San Diego, School of Medicine.

Marc A. Schuckit is Professor, Department of Psychiatry, University of California, San Diego, School of Medicine, and Director, Alcohol and Drug Treatment Program /Alcohol Research Center, San Diego Veterans Affairs Medical Center.

Correspondence should be addressed to Robert M. Anthenelli, MD, Psychiatry Service (116-A), Veterans Affairs Medical Center, 3350 La Jolla Village Drive, San Diego, CA 92161.

This work was supported by the Veterans Affairs Research Service, a VA Psychiatry Research Training Fellowship, and NIAAA Grants #05526, #08401 and #08403.

[Haworth co-indexing entry note]: "Affective and Anxiety Disorders and Alcohol and Drug Dependence: Diagnosis and Treatment." Anthenelli, Robert M., and Marc A. Schuckit. Co-published simultaneously in *Journal of Addictive Diseases,* (The Haworth Press, Inc.) Vol. 12, No. 3, 1993, pp. 73-87; and: *Comorbidity of Addictive and Psychiatric Disorders* (Ed: Norman S. Miller, and Barry Stimmel) The Haworth Press, Inc., 1993, pp. 73-87. Multiple copies of this article/chapter may be purchased from The Haworth Document Delivery Center. Call 1-800-3-HAWORTH (1-800-342-9678) between 9:00 - 5:00(EST) and ask for DOCUMENT DELIVERY CENTER.

to have a different course and prognosis than uncomplicated, independent anxiety and major depressive disorders, and clinicians
should consider the role of alcohol and other drugs in all patients
presenting with these complaints. The authors also outline an approach for diagnosing and managing patients with the combination of
a substance use and depressive or anxiety disorder.

INTRODUCTION

Patients present for help with problems and it is the clinician's
task to sort through these complaints and make the appropriate
diagnosis. When the patient describes a constellation of symptoms
and signs, or syndrome, that fits neatly under a single diagnostic
label, the doctor or therapist is usually well-versed in how to manage the individual with the appropriate treatment. The job becomes
considerably more challenging, however, when the symptoms are
occurring in the setting of heavy alcohol or other drug use.

These substances can mimic symptoms and signs of nearly all of
the major psychiatric syndromes.[1-3] Confounding this further is that
substance-abusing patients seldom volunteer information about
their alcohol and drug use patterns when they present their psychological complaints, and that the co-occurrence of a psychiatric and
substance problem is more likely to bring the individual into the
clinic seeking help.[4] Unless asked about their use of drugs, the
patient's denial and minimization of her/his substance-related problems will keep this important information hidden, making proper
diagnosis and treatment more difficult.

Two of the most common comorbid conditions in alcoholics and
drug abusers are anxiety and depression. There are several factors
contributing to this. First, substance use, anxiety, and depressive
disorders are among the most prevalent psychiatric diagnoses in the
general population.[5] According to data from the ECA study, it is
estimated that about 5 to 15% of individuals will develop alcoholism at some point in their lifetime; anxiety syndromes including
phobic, panic, and obsessive-compulsive disorders are seen in
about the same percentage across the life-span; and about 5 to 10%
of men and women will suffer a major depressive episode at some
point during their lives.[4] Because there is no evidence that having
one of these disorders protects an individual from suffering a second

illness, then minimally one should see dual diagnosis (i.e., a major psychiatric illness and a substance use disorder) rates in the general population occurring at a base rate consistent with that of the most prevalent single disorder.

Second, there is a complex relationship between anxiety and depressive disorders on the one hand, and substance use disorders on the other, which remains the topic of active inquiry. All substances of abuse cross the blood-brain barrier and produce changes in mood and behavior.[3] These alterations occur in a variety of conditions. For example, *intoxication* with brain stimulants (cocaine, amphetamine, etc.) can produce signs and symptoms of anxiety with anxious mood, rapid heart rate and, at higher doses, even panic attacks. Similar symptom patterns may be produced during the *withdrawal* phase from alcohol and other brain depressants, while intoxication with these agents can cause sadness that, when it occurs in the setting of heavy prolonged use, might even take on the proportions of a major depression with changes in mood, self-attitude, and psychovegetative state. But unlike the major psychiatric illnesses specified in the DSM-III R as major depression, generalized anxiety disorder, or panic disorder, these substance-related conditions appear to have different courses, prognoses and treatment needs with most improving or completely resolving within weeks of stopping the drugs. Thus, it is important for clinicians to include an evaluation of patients' drug and alcohol histories in every evaluation of complaints of anxiety and depression and to devise a scheme with which individuals presenting with multiple problems can be evaluated in a way most likely to arrive at the correct diagnosis.

One such approach with both practical and heuristic implications is to determine primary versus secondary diagnoses based on the chronology of development of symptoms.[1-3,6] Using this technique, the "primary" disorder is the symptom cluster which appeared first in the patient's clinical history. For instance, if an individual developed multiple, major life problems because of her/his repeated use of alcohol before the onset of any major psychiatric illness, then that person is most likely to run the course of "primary alcoholism" or alcohol dependence with additional psychiatric symptomatology subsumed under a "secondary" classification.[1,3] Conversely, patients exhibiting bipolar disorder who then later go on to develop alcohol-related life problems (so-called "secondary alcoholics") will most likely follow the course typified by manic-depressive illness with episodic mood swings requiring treatment with mood stabilizers. More than just a research technique, this scheme has clinical implications with data from our laboratory and others showing that secondary diagnoses in drug-abusing patients have their own unique course, prognosis, and treatment needs which differ from the textbook, "single disorder" treatment approach.[7,8]

This clinically-oriented paper examines the relationship between anxiety, depression and substance use disorders. Because most data are from studies in alcoholics, this drug will be emphasized and we will only briefly discuss the relationship between these states and stimulant, opiate, and cannabinol abuse (see references 3, 9-10 for more comprehensive reviews of these topics). We will first highlight some information regarding the interaction between acute and chronic alcohol use and these common psychiatric presentations, and then discuss some general guidelines useful in the diagnosis and management of these complicated patients.

DEPRESSION AND ALCOHOL AND DRUG DEPENDENCE

Symptoms are not diagnoses. Discussions about the relationship between alcoholism, drug abuse and depressed mood often ignore this distinction resulting in a broad range of estimates on the rates of "depression" among alcoholics and drug addicts. Although discussed in greater detail in previous articles,[1,11] this section briefly reviews some of the reasons for this diagnostic confusion and then offers some clinical suggestions on managing these patients.

The Interaction Between Drinking, Alcoholism and Depressed Mood

As a typical member of the brain depressant category (along with benzodiazepines and barbiturates), alcohol is capable of producing feelings of sadness.[1,3,11-12] This dysphoria worsens at higher dose ranges or as the blood alcohol concentration falls, and a number of studies in alcoholics have demonstrated that these mood changes occur despite expectations that the drug will have mood elevating effects.[1,11,13] In addition to these "direct" depressant effects, the life stress caused by ethanol misuse and its impact on the alcoholic's lifestyle (e.g., difficulties with relationships, employment and legal problems, etc.) can be so demoralizing that many individuals will seek psychiatric help for "depression." But cross-sectional evaluations of depressive *symptoms* in alcoholics can lead to inflated estimates of the co-occurrence of these two conditions, with estimates using self-report data in recently detoxified alcoholics reaching staggering proportions of up to 98%.[2]

Heavy, prolonged use of alcohol can produce serious states of depression, but there is consistent evidence that these mood changes are likely to improve markedly with abstinence.[1,3,14] For example, in our own laboratory, a study of 191 carefully diagnosed primary alcoholic inpatients revealed that even after more than a week of abstinence, 42% of the subjects had a Hamilton Depression Rating Scale score which fell in the moderately to severely depressed range.[14] However, with the supportive treatment provided on the alcoholism rehabilitation unit and continued abstinence alone, the percentage of subjects endorsing Hamilton scores above 20 dropped to 12% by week two and only 6% by week four. Interestingly, a subsequent follow-up of these men three months after discharge demonstrated no increased recurrence rates in depressive symptoms except among those individuals who returned to the abuse of alcohol or other drugs. These data underscore the notion that the course of these "*secondary* depressions" differs from the usual path of an uncomplicated major depressive episode with most symptoms melting away without treatment with antidepressant medications within 2 to 4 weeks.[4,14]

Thus, the rate of depressive *symptoms* in alcoholics is apt to be quite high depending on the sample selected, the stringency of the criteria used, the time frame in which subjects are studied (i.e., recently detoxified versus after weeks or months of sobriety), and the duration over which the co-occurrence of symptoms is evaluated (in the last month or over a lifetime). Limiting the definition of depression to more syndromic proportions and including only persistent affective disturbances which interfere with functioning over a period of two or more weeks, about one third of alcoholics suffer severe depressions at some point in their drinking careers.[1,11] However, it appears that after two to four weeks of abstinence, perhaps only 5% of men and about 10% of women with alcoholism are likely to still warrant the diagnosis of a major depressive episode [11]–a rate similar to that of depression in the general population.

The relationship between depression and alcoholism has been examined from other perspectives as well. First, on a genetic level, there remains the question of whether depression and alcoholism are related disorders with shared inheritance. As discussed in other sections of this issue, genetic studies of these two disorders have provided conflicting results, with some investigations demonstrating an increased crossover for alcoholism and depressive disorder within families while others have found little relationship.[11] The latter support the notion that substance-related depression may be a separate phenomenon from major depression.

Second, some controversy remains as to whether individuals "self-medicate" their depressive disorders with alcohol. A throwback to psychiatry's earlier views of alcoholism as a "symptom,"[2] there is little hard evidence supporting this contention. For example, although there are data showing that during the manic phase of bipolar disorder some patients increase their drinking, to the contrary, 70% to 80% of patients with severe depression do not markedly increase their alcohol consumption.[1,11] Similarly, experimental intoxication studies in both normal drinkers and alcoholics consistently show that this drug increases dysphoric feelings rather than alleviating them.[1,11,13] Regardless of the ultimate validity of the self-medication hypothesis, it is essential that the doctor or therapist conveys to the patient that alcohol and other drugs of abuse are not "antidepressants" (the realization that most patients arrive at from their own experience), and that even in individuals with both an independent depressive and substance use disorder, both the alcoholism and depression must be treated.

In summary, although depressive symptoms are a frequent byproduct of heavy drinking, using more stringent criteria it appears that about one third of alcoholics will suffer a severe depression at some point in their drinking career. The majority of these secondary depressions will improve with supportive treatment and abstinence alone. However, there remains a significant minority of patients who will present with both an independent substance use and depressive disorder. In the next sections we briefly discuss the relationship between other drugs of abuse and depression and then describe how the clinician can begin to disentangle these issues and outline a plan for managing these patients.

Depression and Other Drugs of Abuse

In addition to the brain depressants, stimulant (e.g., cocaine and amphetamine) abuse is also frequently associated with affective disturbances. These symptoms predominate during the withdrawal phase when perhaps as many as 50% or more of stimulant abusers are affected.[3,19] As with alcohol-related depressions there is evidence that these mood changes are likely to decrease in intensity within two to four weeks of abstinence. However, some authors suggest a more aggressive approach using psychotropic agents (e.g., desipramine, dopamine agonists, etc.) to ameliorate the marked anhedonia which typifies the "crash" phase of cocaine withdrawal in an effort to decrease craving for the drug and facilitate abstinence.[10,15]

Opiate dependence is also associated with high rates of depressive disorders. Lifetime prevalence rates of depression among opiate addicts and individuals on methadone maintenance approximate 50% to 70% in most patient samples seeking treatment.[9] Similarly, although less data are available, affective disturbances are also reported to be more common during repeated, heavy intoxication with cannabinols.[3]

Managing the Patient with Drug Dependence and Depressive Disorders

With clinical experience and some knowledge of the empirical studies done primarily in patients with alcoholism and depression, the management of patients with comorbid sadness and substance use disorders can be simplified. First, regardless of the primary diagnosis, alcoholics or other substance abusers presenting with depression and suicidal ideation should be considered an emergency situation. Ample data demonstrate the increased prevalence of suicides in alcoholics and drug abusers and the lethality of this combination.[2,3] Therefore, regardless of the clinical setting in which these patients present, the primary/secondary distinction is not an essential part in the decision-making process regarding hospitalization of the suicidal individual.[1]

Second, it is very important to gather the history from both the patient and a resource person (usually a spouse, other relative, or close friend).[1] This is especially helpful in substance-abusing patients because alcoholics and drug abusers are liable to minimize their substance-related problems, because certain drugs (e.g., brain depressants) are more likely to impair memory in these patients making history-taking less reliable, and because the clinician has few options other than a careful clinical history to make the proper diagnosis. Although more time-consuming and still far from perfect, the resource person interview is especially useful in establishing patterns of alcohol and drug use, their relationship to psychologic symptoms, and their time course. Similarly, once the patient's permission has been obtained, this interview can open the door on some of the broader effects that alcohol and drugs are having on the family and can assist in developing the therapeutic alliance.

During these interviews, the clinician should try to distinguish between symptoms and syndromes, consider their duration and severity, and establish the context in which they occur. For example, it would be inappropriate to label an individual as having a major depression if the mood changes appeared only during periods of intoxication or withdrawal or if they were of insufficient severity and duration to warrant such a diagnosis. An analogy can be drawn to bereavement when, in the setting of the recent loss, an individual will experience sadness, grief, and even evidence some vegetative signs but the course and prognosis for these psychologic problems differ from those of a frank major depressive episode.

If it is determined that the patient probably does have two or more diagnoses, then one helpful approach is to attempt to establish a time line of the patient's life. This reconstruction of the clinical history allows one to disentangle the time course of the disorders and helps establish primary versus secondary diagnoses. Rather than focusing on the age when the patient first drank or the time she or he first got intoxicated, instead, the age at which the patient first fulfilled criteria for alcoholism or drug abuse is noted. One short-hand method to approximate this is by noting the first time that alcohol or drug use had actually interfered in a major way in a relationship, the first time an individual had received treatment for alcoholism or drug abuse or was told that drugs had harmed her/his life, the age of a second arrest for alcohol or drugs, and so on. Similarly, psychiatric symptoms and signs are reviewed across the life-span. Recollection of the chronology of the appearance of these problems can be enhanced by framing the interview around impor-tant landmarks in time (e.g., the year the patient graduated high school, his/her wedding date, military discharge date, etc.). Not only does this method help ensure the most accurate chronological reconstruction of the patient's problems, but also, on a therapeutic level, this review helps patients see the relationship between their substance abuse and psychologic symptoms and begins to address some of the denial mechanisms which tend to keep these associa-tions out of mind.

Throughout this process it is important to probe for any periods of abstinence that the patient may have had, noting whether this affected the patient's mood problems. A conservative approach is to establish periods of abstinence lasting 2 to 3 months because it is common for at least some mood changes and psychovegetative signs to persist in a protracted manner in some alcoholics and drug abusers.[1] Then, after reviewing the time line, primary and second-ary diagnoses are determined. Major depressive episodes which occurred before the onset of alcoholism or drug abuse or which were observed during periods of total abstinence lasting several months or more most likely point to the possibility that the patient suffers two disorders (i.e., primary depression with secondary alco-holism). Conversely, if no major psychiatric syndrome can be docu-mented either before the approximate age of onset of alcoholism or drug abuse or during periods of prolonged abstinence, then it is likely that the patient has primary alcoholism or drug abuse and that the depression is secondary.

Finally, the clinician must remain flexible with this working diagnosis and continue to closely observe the patient over time. Like most psychiatric diagnoses which rely so heavily on obtaining complex clinical histories this scheme is hardly foolproof, and even the best efforts at determining primary versus secondary status will be wrong about 5% to 10% of the time. Clearly, an individual who appears to have primary alcoholism with a secondary major depressive disorder but who remains suicidal and morbidly depressed after 4 weeks of abstinence, probably does indeed have an independent major depression requiring aggressive treatment. Similarly, it is important to follow the patients' course even if there is improvement with abstinence and supportive treatment alone during the first weeks of sobriety to ensure that mood symptoms which are liable to appear during this difficult adjustment period do not require other interventions beyond those offered in standard substance abuse treatment programs.

Common sense and some knowledge of the data emerging from empirical studies indicating the relatively rapid improvement in depressive symptoms in most primary alcoholics with abstinence alone dictates that antidepressant medications be used cautiously in this population. We usually advise a 2 to 4 week observation period before considering the use of these medications, emphasizing instead supportive and cognitive/behavioral treatments. This conservative approach ensures that the patient will not be needlessly committed to a 6 to 9 month course of unnecessary pharmacotherapy, minimizes the risk of potential drug interactions, and takes into consideration that there is little convincing evidence that the standard antidepressant medications are effective in the treatment of alcohol-related mood changes. When antidepressant medications are indicated as in the case of the abstinent alcoholic with an independent major depressive episode, careful consideration of the patient's health status should be made.

ANXIETY AND ALCOHOL AND DRUG DEPENDENCE

Many of the comments made regarding the relationship between depressive and substance use disorders are applicable to the discussion of anxiety, alcoholism and drug abuse. To avoid redundancy, in this section we highlight data examining the course of secondary anxiety disorders and touch on some of the issues involved in the complex interaction between abuse of substances and anxiety disorders.

The Interaction Between Drinking, Alcoholism, and Anxiety

There are several reasons why anxiety symptoms and drinking problems frequently coexist in patients prompting them to seek help. First, as mentioned previously, symptoms of anxiety abound during the acute and protracted withdrawal states following periods of heavy alcohol intake. As was the case for depressive symptoms, if one measures the occurrence of these symptoms among recently detoxified or even newly sober (e.g., perhaps following 2 to 3 months of abstinence) alcoholics, almost all of these individuals will experience signs and symptoms of anxiety.[1,16,17] For example, in a recent investigation of 171 male inpatients with primary alcoholism, 98% had experienced multiple symptoms of mild anxiety during withdrawal, and 80% reported shortness of breath or cardiac awareness soon after stopping drinking, including 40% with both somatic complaints.[16] However, the course of these secondary anxiety symptoms improved with abstinence and supportive and behavioral techniques alone during the month-long index hospitalization. Whereas 40% of these men scored in the 75th percentile or higher on the Spielberger State Anxiety Inventory (STAI) scale during their first week of abstinence, by week two the self-report anxiety measures returned to within the normal range for the vast majority.[18] Similarly, at 3-months follow-up, the 41% of alcoholics who had returned to drinking were more likely to show elevated scores on the STAI with only 5% of the abstainers scoring above the 75th precentile on this measure.[18] Thus, secondary anxiety *symptoms* are common during the acute and protracted withdrawal phase of heavy drinking, but have a different course and response to treatment than do primary anxiety disorders.

Second, there remains an active interest in better understanding the relationship between anxiety disorders and the possibility that individuals might "self-medicate" their symptoms with ethanol. Proponents of this hypothesis cite high rates of alcoholism in some groups of psychiatric patients with anxiety disorders;[19] increased levels of anxiety during withdrawal in alcoholics with a co-existing anxiety disorder compared to alcoholics without a second diagnosis;[20] and an increased prevalence of alcoholism among close relatives of individuals with panic disorder.[19] Reflecting the complexity of this issue and the scope of this clinically-oriented discussion, the interested reader is referred to more comprehensive reviews on these topics;[16,17] however, for our purposes, several comments do bear mentioning.

Realizing that symptoms of anxiety and alcoholism go hand in hand and that the relationship between the disorders is complex and not yet fully understood, efforts at establishing primary versus secondary distinctions of these conditions has clinical relevance. There are a number of lines of evidence consistent with the probability that anxiety and substance use disorders are usually discrete diagnoses as was the case for alcoholism and depression.[1,16,17] As the data presented above indicate, there is emerging evidence that when anxiety occurs in the setting of heavy alcohol or other drug use that the course of these secondary disorders tend to be self-limited in contrast to the major anxiety disorders themselves. Similarly, family and genetic studies of alcoholism and anxiety provide conflicting results. In our own laboratory, comparisons of anxiety scores and diagnoses of anxiety disorders in sons of alcoholics with scores from matched controls showed no increased prevalence of either anxiety symptoms or diagnoses in the group at high risk for alcoholism.[17] Combining this with the results of adoption and long-term follow-up studies demonstrating no firm link between anxiety and alcoholism, there is little consistent evidence to indicate a very high rate of independent anxiety disorders among alcoholics.

Anxiety and Other Drugs of Abuse

In addition to ethanol, all brain depressant drugs (e.g., benzodiazepines, barbiturates, etc.) are likely to produce anxiety symptoms during acute and protracted withdrawal. When these drugs have been taken in high enough doses for a sufficient period of time their acute withdrawal might induce panic attacks and phobic symptoms. Although the majority of these signs and symptoms usually improve within the first week or two of abstinence, many signs such as changes in autonomic nervous system functioning and sleep disturbances may persist in a diminished form for up to several months.[3,17]

As mentioned earlier, intoxication with stimulants (e.g., cocaine and amphetamines) can also produce marked symptoms and signs of anxiety including feelings of nervousness, palpitations, and even frank panic attacks.[3] Individuals abusing these drugs may present with complaints which resemble generalized anxiety, panic, or obsessive-compulsive disorder.[3,17] However, as described above, if the anxiety developed in the setting of heavy drug abuse, symptoms are likely to improve with abstinence alone.

Physically dependent stimulant abusers exhibit numerous symptoms of anxiety, usually mixed with depression, during the withdrawal phase. Although the majority of these problems improve over the first two to four weeks, occasionally some individuals experience a more protracted course over several months.[3] Finally, cannabinols (marijuana, hashish, etc.) are capable of producing intense but temporary feelings of anxiety and panic-like states during acute intoxication.[3]

Managing the Patient with Drug Dependence and Anxiety Disorders

The general guidelines described in the previous section on drug abuse and depression apply to the patient presenting with a combination of anxiety and substance-related complaints.[1,17] Again, with the help of a resource person, we find it is possible to reconstruct the patient's substance-related and psychological problems on a time line emphasizing the diagnosis of syndromes and not just symptoms. When anxiety disorders are seen either before the onset of alcohol-related life problems or during an abstinence period of 2 to 3 months, then it is likely that the patient might have two disorders, each of which may require treatment.

But if the anxiety symptoms occur almost exclusively in the setting of heavy alcohol or other drug intake, then it is likely that the anxiety is secondary to the substance abuse and that it will improve with the combination of abstinence and supportive and behavioral measures, showing signs of improvement within the first 2 to 4 weeks.

Regardless of our initial working diagnosis, we always carefully observe the patient over time and reevaluate her/his condition. With this approach, one avoids missing the possibility that the patient has two independent disorders requiring more aggressive treatment. However, at the same time, this approach decreases the chance that medications are started prematurely when indeed the course of the disorder would be to show improvement with sobriety alone.

Even in individuals with an independent or primary anxiety disorder, it is important to educate the patient that alcohol and other drug use only makes their condition worse and that these agents are equally poor as long-term anxiolytics as they were as antidepressants. In treating patients with anxiety and substance use disorders, the mainstay of treatment rests with education, supportive therapy, and cognitive/behavioral techniques (see ref. 17 for a more comprehensive discussion). As was the case for depressive disorders, medications should be used sparingly; however, patients with independent anxiety disorders might require pharmacotherapy in addition to counseling.

REFERENCES

1. Schuckit MA, Monteiro MG. Alcoholism, anxiety and depression. Br J Addict. 1988;83:1373-1380.

2. Solomon J. Alcoholism and psychiatric disorders. In: Goedde HW, Agarwal PD, eds. Alcoholism: Biomedical and genetic aspects. New York: Pergamon Press, 1989:216-227.

3. Schuckit MA. Drug and alcohol abuse: A clinical guide to diagnosis and treatment. 3rd ed. New York: Plenum Medical Book Company, 1989.

4. Helzer JE, Pryzbeck TR. The co-occurrence of alcoholism with other psychiatric disorders in the general population and its impact on treatment. J Stud Alcohol 1988;49:219-224.

5. Regier DA, Boyd JH, Burke JD, et al. One-month prevalence of mental disorders in the United States: Based on five Epidemiologic Catchment Area sites. Arch Gen Psychiatry 1988;45:977-986.

6. Goodwin DW, Guze SB. Psychiatric diagnosis. 4th ed. New York: Oxford University Press, 1989.

7. Schuckit MA. The clinical implications of primary diagnostic groups among alcoholics. Arch Gen Psychiatry 1985;42:1043-1049.

8. Powell BJ, Read MR, Penick EC, et al. Primary and secondary depression in alcoholic men: An important distinction? J Clin Psychiatry 1987;48:98-101.

9. Rounsaville BJ, Weissman MM, Kleber H, et al. Heterogeneity of psychiatric diagnosis in treated opiate addicts. Arch Gen Psychiatry 1982; 39: 161-166.

10. Gawin FH, Ellinwood EH. Cocaine and other stimulants: Actions, abuse, and treatment. N Engl J Med 1988;318:1173-1182.

11. Schuckit MA. Genetic and clinical implications of alcoholism and affective disorder. Am J Psychiatry 1986;143:140-147.

12. Anthenelli RM, Schuckit MA. Alcohol and cerebral depressants. In: Glass IB, ed. The international handbook of addiction behaviour. London: Routledge Publishers; 1991.

13. Tamerin JS, Weiner S, Mendelson JH. Alcoholics' expectancies and recall of experiences during intoxication. Am J Psychiatry 1970;126:1697-1704.

14. Brown SA, Schuckit MA. Changes in depression among abstinent alcoholics. J Stud Alcohol 1988;49:412-417.

15. Gawin FH, Kleber HD, Byck R, et al. Desipramine facilitation of initial cocaine abstinence. Arch Gen Psychiatry 1989;46:117-121.

16. Schuckit MA, Irwin M, Brown SA. The history of anxiety symptoms among 171 primary alcoholics. J Stud Alcohol 1990;51:34-41.

17. Schuckit MA. Treatment of anxiety in patients who abuse alcohol and drugs. In: Noyes Jr. R, Roth M, Burrows GD, eds. Handbook of anxiety, Vol. 4: The treatment of anxiety. Elsevier Science Publishers B.V., 1990.

18. Brown SA, Irwin M, Schuckit MA. Changes in anxiety among abstinent male alcoholics. J Stud Alcohol 1991;52:55-61.

19. Weissman M. Anxiety and alcoholism. J Clin Psychiatry 1988;49(10S): 17-19.

20. Thevkos AK, Johnston AL, Latham PK, et al. Symptoms of anxiety in inpatient alcoholics with and without DSM-III-R anxiety disorders. Alcohol Clin Exp Res 1991;15:102-105.

Pathological Gambling, Eating Disorders, and the Psychoactive Substance Use Disorders

Henry R. Lesieur, PhD
Sheila B. Blume, MD

SUMMARY. Both pathological gambling and the eating disorders have been conceptualized as addictive diseases, comparable to alcoholism and other drug dependencies. This paper briefly reviews both pathological gambling and the eating disorders, stressing their epidemiology and their overlap with psychoactive substance use and other psychiatric disorders. Common factors in the natural history and treatment of these disorders are also discussed.

Henry R. Lesieur is Professor and Chair, Department of Criminal Justice Sciences, Illinois State University, Normal, IL.

Sheila B. Blume is Medical Director, South Oaks Hospital, Amityville, New York, and Clinical Professor of Psychiatry, State University of New York at Stony Brook, Stony Brook, NY.

Reprint requests should be addressed to Henry R. Lesieur, PhD, South Oaks Institute of Alcoholism and Addictive Behavior Studies, 400 Sunrise Highway, Amityville, NY 11701.

[Haworth co-indexing entry note]: "Pathological Gambling, Eating Disorders, and the Psychoactive Substance Use Disorders." Lesieur, Henry R., and Sheila B. Blume. Co-published simultaneously in *Journal of Addictive Diseases*, (The Haworth Press, Inc.) Vol. 12, No. 3, 1993, pp. 89-102; and: *Comorbidity of Addictive and Psychiatric Disorders* (Ed: Norman S. Miller, and Barry Stimmel) The Haworth Press, Inc., 1993, pp. 89-102. Multiple copies of this article/chapter may be purchased from The Haworth Document Delivery Center. Call 1-800-3-HAWORTH (1-800-342-9678) between 9:00 - 5:00(EST) and ask for DOCUMENT DELIVERY CENTER.

89

INTRODUCTION

In his extensive review of the relevant historical and clinical literature, Orford compares alcoholism, dependence on other drugs (including nicotine), compulsive gambling, excessive eating and excessive sexuality.[1] This comparison is used to formulate a general psychological model of addiction. In addition to these five categories of excessive behavior, anorexia nervosa has also been conceptualized as an addictive disorder.[2] One factor common to the drugs and behaviors that develop into addictions in some individuals is their potential for producing pleasure, or at least relief from painful emotional states. However, other pleasurable, stress-reducing behaviors (for example: reading, gardening or playing a musical instrument) seldom, if ever, seem to evolve into addiction-like behavior patterns. Future research may well establish that the link to the addictive pattern is a neurochemical one. It may be that these "addictive" behaviors are able (at least in predisposed individuals) to stimulate the endogenous production of opiates, psycho-stimulants or other analogs of the exogenous substances which have high addiction potential. For example, elevated levels of opioids have been reported in studies of anorexia, bulimia and obesity,[2] while elevated levels of norepinephrine metabolites have been found in compulsive gamblers.[3] Recovering compulsive gamblers have described their disorder as being "hooked on their own adrenalin."

In addition to considerations of possible neurochemical mechanisms, the various addictions share the importance of sociocultural factors in their development. The long history of social controls of alcohol and other drug use are parallelled by controls on gambling. Over the course of history and around the world the human race has seen fit to regulate, criminalize, decriminalize and legalize both the whole range of psychoactive substances and various forms of gambling.[4,5] Such measures have drastically influenced the availability of these substances and of wagering opportunities, which in turn has affected the probability that any individual in a particular society will be sufficiently exposed to the substance (or to gambling) to initiate addictive behavior. The current United States "war on drugs" has sought to reduce the overall availability and acceptability of the "illegal" drugs. At the same time, attempts are being made to increase enforcement of control laws, increase taxes and promote public education about the dangers of excessive drinking and of smoking. However, the opposite trend is apparent in gambling, with the increasing legalization of lotteries, sports betting and casino gambling during the past two decades. Today Americans gamble for God (bingo, "Las Vegas Nites," raffles and punchboards) and Country (state-run lotteries and taxes on the proceeds of privately-operated games). This increase in availability and acceptability will almost surely lead to an increase in gambling problems.

Our relationship to food is also culturally mediated. In societies where starvation is common, fat is praised as a sign of wealth and health. In prosperous industrialized societies, fat is seen as unnecessary baggage. Also within industrial societies the relation to food differs between the sexes. Males are granted more latitude in weight than females, who have been barraged with the cult of thinness and the visual objectification of women.[6] In America, for example, over the past three decades cosmetic ideals of female body shape have gotten thinner.[7] This has had the effect of producing eating disorders (namely anorexia nervosa and bulimia) in Western societies which are virtually unknown in places like the People's Republic of China.[8]

PATHOLOGICAL GAMBLING

The American Psychiatric Association (1987) defines pathological gambling as a chronic and progressive failure to resist impulses to gamble, and gambling behavior that compromises, disrupts, or damages personal, family, or vocational pursuits.[9] Problem gamblers are individuals who exhibit some signs of pathological gambling but are not sufficiently symptomatic to meet the full diagnosis.

While pathological gambling does not involve the use of a substance, research conducted by numerous scholars has noted its similarity to addictive behaviors.[3] For example, pathological gamblers characteristically state that what they seek is "action" (often more important than money or escape from problems). The term refers to an aroused, euphoric state comparable to the "high" derived from cocaine or other drugs.[3] Action means excitement, thrills and tension, "when the adrenalin is flowing." The desire to remain in action is so intense that many gamblers will go for days without sleep, eating or using the bathroom. Being in action pushes out all other concerns. There is also a "rush," usually characterized by nervousness, excitement, sweaty palms and rapid heart beat, which is experienced during the period of anticipation.

Pathological gamblers, like alcoholics and drug addicts, are frequently preoccupied with seeking out gambling; they gamble longer than intended and with more money than intended. There is also the equivalent of "tolerance," described in race track, sports, and casino bettors[3] who state they could no longer get excited by small bets once they were making large wagers. Further investigation is needed relative to slot and poker machine gambling. Self-reported withdrawal symptoms have been the subject of several studies[10] which have documented the equivalent of both psychological and psychosomatic withdrawal symptoms in pathological gamblers who stop gambling.

Like alcohol, drug and food addicts, pathological gamblers frequently try to cut down and quit their addiction. While gambling does not produce the cognitive or physical impairment characteristic of alcohol or drug intoxication, the obsession with gambling has been noted to impair performance in personal, social and occupational functioning.

"Dimensions" for each of the diagnostic criteria for the proposed DSM-IV are: (1) progression and preoccupation, (2) tolerance, (3) withdrawal, (4) use of gambling as an escape, (5) chasing losses, (6) lies/deception, (7) illegal acts, (8) family/job disruption, (9) need for a financial bailout, and (10) loss of control.

EPIDEMIOLOGY OF PATHOLOGICAL GAMBLING

Available evidence suggests that where more forms of gambling are legal, there is a higher incidence of pathological gambling. In 1974, fewer than one percent of the U.S. adult population were recognized as compulsive gamblers while the comparable rate for Nevada was 2.5%.[11] More recently, surveys have been done in New York, New Jersey, Maryland, and Iowa in the U.S. and Quebec, Canada.[3,12-14] These studies revealed that the prevalence of problem and pathological gambling in Iowa, where there is less legalized gambling, was about half of that in the other U.S. states studied and Quebec (2% in Iowa versus 4% elsewhere for combined pathological and problem gambling).

These surveys also indicate that the prevalence is greater for males, the poor and minorities than for other segments of the population. There is also evidence that the poor, minorities, and women are grossly underserved by available treatment resources.[3,12] Studies of high school[15] and college students[16] show that rates of probable pathological gambling are three times higher than comparable rates for adults (4% to 6% compared with 1% to 2%).

PSYCHIATRIC DISORDERS
AMONG PATHOLOGICAL GAMBLERS

Pathological gambling overlaps with a variety of psychiatric disorders. In two studies of male inpatients and Gamblers Anonymous (GA) members,[3] 72-76% of the subjects were diagnosed as having major depressive disorder or hypomanic disorder. There was a high rate (20%) of panic disorders in one study as well. In addition, studies have reported rates of suicide attempts by male and female G.A. members and hospitalized male pathological gamblers ranging from 15% to 24%.[3]

One recent study of hospitalized psychiatric patients found that seven of 105 patients surveyed (6.5%) were pathological gamblers.[17] This is a rate four times higher than for the general population.

PATHOLOGICAL GAMBLING
AND PSYCHOACTIVE SUBSTANCE USE DISORDERS

Systematic studies of pathological gamblers have revealed rates of alcohol and other substance use, dependence and abuse ranging from 47% to 52%.[3]

Investigations of patients in substance dependence treatment have found that 9% to 14% could be diagnosed as pathological gamblers and an additional 9% to 14% as problem gamblers.[3,18] These rates are 6 to 10 times higher than for the general population. Pathological gambling appears to compound the already high personal and social costs of substance use disorders, increasing the risk of incarceration,[3] stress-related diseases and serious psychiatric problems including suicide attempts.[3]

EATING DISORDERS

Eating disorders, like pathological gambling, are included in the Diagnostic and Statistical Manual of the American Psychiatric Association.[9] Anorexia nervosa is characterized by an intense fear of becoming fat in spite of being 15% or more below normal weight. It includes self-starvation, a distorted body image, and amenorrhea in females. Self-induced vomiting and/or laxative/diuretic abuse may also be present, and the disease is fatal in between 5% and 18% of cases.[9]

Bulimia nervosa is a related disorder which includes frequent binge eating, feelings of lack of control over eating while on binges, and efforts to prevent weight gain which encompass one or more of the following: self-induced vomiting, laxative or diuretic abuse, strict dieting or fasting, and excessive exercise. In common with anorexia nervosa there is an obsession with body weight.

Obesity itself is not strictly an eating disorder since it many have a variety of causes. Compulsive overeating in a pattern of eating binges with loss of control is typically classified as bulimia, or "Eating Disorder Not Otherwise Specified" when not all the diagnostic criteria for bulimia are met.

EPIDEMIOLOGY OF EATING DISORDERS

Surveys of the general population reveal that eating disorders are most common among young, middle class females.[8] In the Epidemiologic Catchment Area survey,[19] the rate of anorexia nervosa was reported to be 0.1% in the general population and the disorder was not found among blacks. Rates of bulimia were not reported. Most of the prevalence studies on bulimia and anorexia have been conducted among young female populations. Rates of bulimia range from 1% to 8% in this group,[8,20] while anorexia is found in slightly less than 1% of schoolgirls studied.[21]

PSYCHIATRIC DISORDERS
AMONG EATING DISORDERED INDIVIDUALS

Psychiatric disorders found at increased rates among bulimic patients include major affective disorders, obsessive-compulsive disorder, and psychoactive substance use disorders.[22] Rates of affective disorder for individuals with bulimia nervosa range from 43% to 88%.[8,23] Obese binge eaters when compared with obese non-binge eaters exhibit more psychiatric disorders, primarily affective disorders, major depression in particular, as measured by the Diagnostic Interview Schedule.[24]

EATING DISORDERS
AND PSYCHOACTIVE SUBSTANCE USE DISORDERS

There is substantial multiple addiction among eating disordered patients, particularly bulimics. Rates for alcohol and other drug dependence appear to increase with age and range from 13% to 22% for high school and college freshmen to 31% to 50% in studies of individuals in their 30s and 40s.[8] Mitchell and colleagues report there are fewer studies of substance use disorders among anorectics but they show lower rates than bulimics.[8]

Studies of alcohol and drug dependent individuals also show patterns of eating disorders. In a study of 259 callers to the cocaine hotline, Jonas and Gold found that 22% fulfilled the DSM-III criteria for bulimia, 7% for both bulimia and anorexia and 2% for anorexia alone.[23] Peveler and Fairburn found 36% of women attending an alcohol treatment unit showed symptoms of binge eating, 26% fulfilled diagnoses of clinical eating disorders, and 19% were anorectic.[25]

COMMONALITIES AMONG PATHOLOGICAL GAMBLING,
EATING DISORDERS, AND SUBSTANCE USE
DISORDERS

Disorders classified as addictions, such as pathological gambling, eating disorders, and psychoactive substance dependence have commonalities, reciprocity, and overlap (see Table 1). Jockeys, for example, are reported to have high rates of both bulimia and pathological gambling. The bulimia is related to their desire to maintain a low

---

Table 1. Addictive Behavior Patterns in Excessive Gambling, Eating, and Drug
Use.

	Pathological Gambling	Eating Disorders	Drug Dependence
Progression	yes	yes	yes
Preoccupation	yes	yes	yes
Loss of Control	yes	yes	yes
Physiological tolerance	no	?	yes (some drugs)
Psychological tolerance	yes	?	yes
Physiological withdrawal	?	no	yes (some drugs)
Psychological withdrawal	yes	?	yes
Health consequences	yes	yes	yes
Family consequences	yes	yes	yes
Occupational consequences	yes	not usually	yes
Financial consequences	yes	no	yes
Legal consequences	yes	no	yes
Arousal	yes	?	yes
Escape	yes	yes	yes
Treatment			
self-help (AA model)	yes	yes	yes
addiction model applied by			
treatment professionals	yes	yes	yes
abstinence	yes	not possible	yes

---

weight while gambling is an occupational exposure which increases the probability of developing gambling-related problems.

Addictions have reciprocity. Engaging in one increases the risk for another. Individuals report gambling, eating, and using drugs for similar reasons, such as relief of anxiety, boredom, and depression.[3,23] These three activities are often engaged in at the same time. Furthermore, patients who suffer from these disorders exhibit similar patterns of affective illness.

While systematic studies of comorbidity between pathological gambling and eating disorders have not been conducted, some research does point to joint occurrence. Lesieur and colleagues, in an inquiry into college student gambling, found that overeating was associated with pathological gambling while "overeating then vomiting" was not.[16] Lesieur and Blume reported that ten out of fifty pathological gambling women interviewed (20%) called themselves compulsive overeaters while another had been anorectic in her youth.[26] One of these women reported leaving work and searching out card games with the best food, gorging herself prior to the game, and then not eating until the game ended, sometimes ten to fifteen hours later. Another of the subjects preferred to prepare food for hours prior to card games she ran at her own home. Food was central to superstitious practices among some of these women as well. Eating was felt to be unlucky for some but lucky for others. Most, however, did not like food at the table during the game itself as it slowed down the action.

The authors analyzed data collected in a recent survey conducted in connection with DSM-IV.[3] This survey involved 209 pathological gamblers in treatment and a control group of 103 substance dependent patients. Subjects were asked if they felt they were "compulsive overeaters or have an eating disorder." Pathological gamblers who were also alcohol or drug dependent were more likely to admit to having an eating disorder than gamblers without substance use disorders or alcohol or drug dependent patients who were not pathological gamblers. We found that 22 (36%) of 61 pathological gamblers with collateral alcohol or drug dependence, 35 (24%) of 148 of pathological gamblers without substance dependence, but just 11 (11%) of 103 substance dependent patients without gambling problems described themselves as having an eating disorder (Cramer's V = .22, chi-square = 15.5, df = 2, p < .001).

Additional parallels among pathological gambling, eating disorders, and alcohol or drug dependence have been described. Hatsukami and colleagues note that both bulimics and psychoactive substance dependent patients exhibit loss of control over food or drugs substance, are secretive about their behavior, and become socially isolated.[23] Similar patterns have been noted for pathological gamblers.[3]

Progression, preoccupation, loss of control and disregard for consequences[3,23] clearly exist among pathological gamblers and binge eaters in ways which approximate these conditions among alcoholic or drug addicted individuals. As the disorder progresses, life problems exacerbate and the behavior, once pleasurable, becomes ego-dystonic. As mentioned above, tolerance and withdrawal have been described in pathological gamblers, although not among eating disorder patients.

In addition to the above phenomena, trance-like, or dissociative states and blackouts among pathological gamblers and compulsive overeaters are described by clinicians and have been the subject of some research.[3,27] However, the exact nature of these phenomena needs further investigation.

As in psychoactive substance use disorders, there are adverse health consequences related to pathological gambling and eating disorders. For pathological gamblers this means heart problems, intestinal disorders, migraine and other stress-related diseases;[28] for bulimics and anorexics this can mean malnutrition, blood chemistry imbalances, and cardiopulmonary, gastrointestinal and dental problems. In addition, there may be medical emergencies produced by induced vomiting, and laxative or diuretic abuse.[8,29]

When we consider the possibility of financial, occupational and legal consequences however, gambling fits the dependence/addiction model more closely than do eating disorders. Pathological gamblers mount up enormous debts, jeopardize their employment, and many become involved in illegal activities in connection with attempts to pay gambling-related debts or to continue gambling.[3,26] There appears to be some association between eating disorders (particularly bulimia) and stealing.[23,30] While many of the bulimics studied stole food, they also reported stealing jewelry and other non-food items for personal use. The psychological mechanisms relating stealing to bulimia have not been delineated, and the relationship remains unclear.

SCREENING SUBSTANCE ABUSERS FOR GAMBLING AND EATING PROBLEMS

Given the relatively high prevalence of eating disorders and pathological gambling among substance abusers it is recommended that all of these patients be screened for gambling and eating problems.

Several screening instruments have been developed for eating disorders, including the Eating Attitudes Test (EAT),[31] and the Eating Disorders Inventory (EDI).[32] These questionnaires measure attitudes and patterns associated with eating disorders. The EAT and EDI are widely used by clinicians to aid in screening of patients for eating disorders.

There is currently only one reliable, validated screening instrument used to identify pathological gamblers, the South Oaks Gambling Screen (the SOGS).[33] The SOGS can be conveniently administered as a pencil and paper test or a structured interview. It is currently in use across the United States and has been translated into a dozen other languages.

TREATMENT STRATEGIES

The psychoactive substance use disorders and pathological gambling may be treated simultaneously,[34] with successful outcome.[3] Eating disorders that co-occur with substance use disorders are often treated sequentially in inpatient programs.[8] However, at South Oaks Hospital, joint treatment plans are often developed between the chemical dependency and eating disorder units, both of which utilize 12-step programs as part of their treatment philosophy.

The phases and goals of treatment are similar in the addictive disorders.[8,35,36] The first phase, intervention, involves initial assessment, problem definition and motivating the patient to enter treatment. In the second phase, the addictive behavior is interrupted, the patient's most threatening immediate problems, including withdrawal symptoms, are addressed and motivational work continues. A more extensive assessment is made and a long term treatment plan developed, including approaches to all related physical, psychiatric, nutritional, interpersonal, occupational, legal and financial aspects of the patient's overall problem. The next phase, rehabilitation, involves educating the patient and family about addictive disorders (including the danger of switching addictions), formulating appropriate strategies to meet life stresses without relapse, developing lasting motivation for continued recovery, teaching healthy patterns of living and linking the patient to an abstinent social support group such as Alcoholics Anonymous, Narcotics Anonymous, Gamblers Anonymous or Overeaters Anonymous. Treatment methods are also similar, including individual, group and family therapies, behavior modification, psychoeducation and specialized counseling (e.g., nutritional, spiritual, financial).

Unfortunately, a final commonality in the current treatment of compulsive gambling and eating disorders is the scarcity of both trained personnel and organized programs for their treatment. Education of professionals, the public, and policy-makers will be necessary to generate sufficient interest and support so that treatment can be made available to all in need.

RESOURCES

Those interested in further information are advised to read two journals: *Journal of Gambling Studies* and the *International Journal of Eating Disorders*. There is a national voluntary association for those interested in gambling problems, the National Council on Problem Gambling. In addition, there are two associations concerned with eating disorders: the National Association of Anorexia, Nervosa and Associated Disorders and the Anorexia/Bulimia Association.[37]

REFERENCES

1. Orford J. Excessive appetites: a psychological view of addictions. Chichester, England: Wiley and Sons, 1985.

2. Jonas JM, Gold MS. Naltrexone treatment of bulimia: clinical and theoretical findings linking eating disorders and substance abuse. Advances in Alcoholism and Substance Abuse, 1988; 7:29-37.

3. Lesieur HR, Rosenthal RJ. Pathological gambling: a review of the literature (prepared for the American Psychiatric Association Task Force on DSM-IV Committee on Disorders of Impulse Control Not Elsewhere Classified). J Gambling Studies, 1991; 7:5-40.

4. Musto DF. The American disease: origins of narcotic control. New York: Oxford University Press, 1987.

5. Rosecrance J. Gambling without guilt: the legitimation of an American pastime. Belmont, CA: Wadsworth Pub., 1988.

6. Schur E. Labeling women deviant: gender, stigma, and social control. New York: Random House, 1984.

7. Fallon AE, Rozin P. Sex differences in perceptions of desirable body shape. J Abnormal Psychology, 1985; 94:102-105.

8. Mitchell JE, Pyle RL, Eckert ED, Specker S. Eating disorders and drug and alcohol addiction. In: Miller N, ed. Handbook of Drug and Alcohol Addiction. New York: Marcel Dekker Inc; in press:193-202.

9. American Psychiatric Association. Diagnostic and statistical manual, third edition, revised. Washington, D.C.: Author, 1987.

10. Rosenthal RJ, Lesieur HR. Self-reported withdrawal symptoms and pathological gambling. Am J Addictions. in press.

11. Kallick M, Suits D, Dielman T, Hybels J. A survey of gambling attitudes and behavior. Ann Arbor, MI: Institute for Social Research, 1987.

12. Volberg RA, Steadman HJ. Prevalence estimates of pathological gambling in New Jersey and Maryland. Am J Psychiatry. 1989; 146: 1618-1619.

13. Volberg RA, Steadman HJ. Prevalence estimates of problem gambling in three states. Remarks presented at the Fourth National Conference on Compulsive Gambling, Des Moines, Iowa, 1989.

14. Ladouceur R. Prevalence estimates of pathological gambling in Quebec. Can J Psychiatry. 1991; 36:732-734.

15. Jacobs DF. Illegal and undocumented: A review of teenage gambling and the plight of children of problem gamblers in America. In: Shaffer HJ, Stein, SA, Gambino B, Cummings TN, eds. Compulsive gambling: theory, research and practice. Lexington, Mass.: Lexington Books, 1989:249-292.

16. Lesieur HR, Cross J, Frank M, Welch M, White C, Rubenstein G, Moseley K, Mark M. Gambling and pathological gambling among college students. Addictive Beh. 1991; 16:517-527.

17. Lesieur HR, Blume SB. Characteristics of pathological gamblers identified among patients on a psychiatric admissions service. Hospital and Community Psychiatry, 1990; 41:1009-1012.

18. Rounsaville BJ, Anton SF, Carroll K, Budde D, Prusoff BA, Gawin F. Psychiatric diagnoses of treatment-seeking cocaine abusers. Arch Gen Psychiatry, 1991; 48:43-51.

19. Robins LN, Helzer JE, Weissman MM, Orvaschel H, Gruenberg E, Burke JD, Regier DA. Lifetime prevalence of specific disorders in three sites. Arch Gen Psychiatry, 1984; 41: 949-958.

20. Hesse-Biber S. Eating patterns and disorders in a college population: Are college women's eating problems a new phenomenon? Sex Roles, 1989; 20:73- 89.

21. Crisp AH, Palmer RL, Kalucy RS. How common is anorexia nervosa? A prevalence study. Brit J Psychiatry, 1976; 128:549-554.

22. Hudson JI, Pope HG, Yurgelun-Todd D, Jonas JM, Frankenburg FR. A controlled study of lifetime prevalence of affective and other psychiatric disorders in bulimic outpatients. Am J Psychiatry, 1987; 144: 1283-1287.

23. Zweben JE. Eating disorders and substance abuse. J Psychoactive Drugs, 1987; 19:181-192.

24. Marcus MD, Wing RR, Ewing L, Kern E, Gooding W, McDermott M. Psychiatric disorders among obese binge eaters. Int J Eating Disorders, 1990; 9:69-77.

25. Peveler R, Fairburn C. Eating disorders in women who abuse alcohol. Brit J Addict, 1990; 85: 1633-1638.

26. Lesieur HR, Blume SB. When lady luck loses: Women and compulsive gambling. In: van den Bergh N, ed. Feminist perspectives on treating addictions. New York: Springer, 1991:181-198.

27. Jacobs DF. Evidence for a common dissociative-like reaction among addicts. J Gambling Beh, 1988; 4:27-37.

28. Lorenz VC, Yaffee RA. Pathological gambling: Psychosomatic, emotional, and marital difficulties as reported by the gambler. J Gambling Beh, 1986; 2:40-49.

29. Riebel L, Kaplan J. Someone you love is obsessed with food. Center City, MN: Hazelden, 1989.

30. McElroy SL, Hudson JI, Pope HG, Keck PE. Kleptomania: Clinical characteristics and associated psychopathology. Psychological Medicine, in press.

31. Garner DM, Olmsted MP, Bohr Y, Garfinkel PE. The eating attitudes test: Psychometric features and clinical correlates. Psychological Medicine, 1982; 12:871-878.

32. Garner DM, Olmsted MP, Polivy J. Development and validation of a multidimensional eating disorder inventory for anorexia nervosa and bulimia. Int J Eating Disorders, 1983; 2: 15-34.

33. Lesieur HR, Blume SB. The South Oaks Gambling Screen (The SOGS): A new instrument for the identification of pathological gamblers. Am J Psychiatry, 1987; 144:1184-1188.

34. Blume SB. Treatment for the addictions: Alcoholism, drug dependence and compulsive gambling in a psychiatric setting. J Substance Abuse Treatment, 1986; 3: 131-133.

35. Blume SB. Alcoholism. In: Conn HF, ed. Current Therapy 1982. Philadelphia, Pa.: W.B. Saunders, 1982: 921-925.

36. Blume SB. Treatment for compulsive gambling. In: Levy SJ, Blume SB, eds. Addictions in the Jewish community. New York: Federation of Jewish Philanthropies, 1986: 371-379.

37. The National Council on Problem Gambling, 445 West 59th Street (Room 1521), New York, NY 10019, (212) 765-3833; National Association of Anorexia Nervosa and Associated Disorders, Highland Park, Illinois 60034, (600) 567-3489; Anorexia/Bulimia Association, 418 E. 76th Street, New York, NY 10021, (212) 734-1114.

The Dually Diagnosed Patient with Psychotic Symptoms

Richard K. Ries, MD

SUMMARY. The dual diagnoses of substance use disorder with other psychiatric disorder is especially problematic in psychotic or other chronically mentally ill patients. Such patients have a more fragile mental status which can be adversely affected by psychoactive substances of abuse. In addition, most such patients need to take potent psychiatric medications which themselves may interact with substances. This article reviews substance induced versus true comorbid major psychiatric disorders and discusses the major classes of psychiatric medications in terms of abuse potential and their abilities to either help or hinder substance disorder recovery.

INTRODUCTION

This discussion will focus on the patient with a concurrence of psychotic symptoms and substance use. The discussion brings informa-

Richard K. Ries is Associate Professor at the Department of Psychiatry and Behavioral Sciences, University of Washington School of Medicine, Seattle, WA.

Correspondence should be addressed to Richard K. Ries, Director, Inpatient Psychiatry, Dual Disorders Programs; Medical Director, Chemical Dependency Project, Harborview Medical Center, 325-9th Avenue, ZA-99, Seattle, WA 98104.

[Haworth co-indexing entry note]: "The Dually Diagnosed Patient with Psychotic Symptoms." Ries, Richard K. Co-published simultaneously in *Journal of Addictive Diseases,* (The Haworth Press, Inc.) Vol. 12, No. 3, 1993, pp. 103-122; and: *Comorbidity of Addictive and Psychiatric Disorders* (Ed: Norman S. Miller, and Barry Stimmel) The Haworth Press, Inc., 1993, pp. 103-122. Multiple copies of this article/chapter may be purchased from The Haworth Document Delivery Center. Call 1-800-3-HAWORTH (1-800-342-9678) between 9:00 - 5:00(EST) and ask for DOCUMENT DELIVERY CENTER.

103

tion to the clinician from two sources: (a) published literature, and (b) clinical experience with running dual diagnosis programs over the last six years. This paper's intent is to blend recent academic information with the perspective of clinical dual diagnosis treatment experience.

I. DIAGNOSIS

It is important to point out that psychotic symptoms may be a (a) result of substance use in a person otherwise not having a psychotic disorder, (b) a result of substance use by a person in which psychotic symptoms may have pre-existed the substance use, or (c) unrelated to substance though pre-existing psychotic symptoms may be increased, altered or even temporarily decreased as a result of the use of substances (i.e., the hallucinating schizophrenic patient whose hallucinations temporarily decrease in intensity as they become inebriated, though symptoms often worsen during the decreasing blood level.)

Some authors[1,2] have attempted to use the primary/secondary distinction in order to characterize whether the psychiatric disorder (example: schizophrenia) or the substance use (example: cocaine) existed first. Other authors[3-5] have largely abandoned the primary/secondary differential, stating that in the clinical forum the historical information needed to establish which came first is usually (a) unavailable, or (b) unreliable, and/or (c) does not often lead to major differential assessment or treatment of the acute patient who has active combined psychosis and substance use, especially if both have been going on for years, as is often the case.

Ries and coworkers[4] have developed a system of defining psychiatric disorder as either low or high in severity depending on severity and persistence of the mental illness. Initial psychiatric severity is assessed in terms of patients ability to perform basic functions and communicate. For example, most psychoses are rated as high severity while most anxiety disorders are rated as low severity. Substance use is characterized on a separate axis which ranges from low (abuse) to high (dependence) in severity depending on whether abuse or dependence is present. Thus patients are categorized on a 2×2 matrix into four categories (1) low psychiatric, low substance, (2) low psychiatric, high substance, (3) high psychiatric/ low substance, (4) high psychiatric/high substance. Most patients with psychotic disorders will be initially classified as high on psychiatric severity and their substance use disorder is classified as high if they meet criteria for substance dependence or low if they meet criteria for substance abuse. Patients with drug induced psychoses might be acutely classified as high in psychiatric severity, however, since most drug induced psychotic symptoms resolve in a few hours or days,[6] these patients would likely be changed from a high psychiatric severity to low or zero psychiatric severity depending on resolution of their psychiatric symptoms. The high/low severity classification system is designed to describe symptom severities which then lead to differential treatment needs, (i.e., patient treatment matching). A more detailed description of the system and its rationale can be found elsewhere.[4]

A. Drug Induced Psychotic Disorders

Probably any drug of abuse, including alcohol, can induce psychotic symptoms if taken in enough quantity or over an extended period of time. We will briefly go through the main drugs and review the most common psychotic symptoms associated with their use or withdrawal.

A.1 Alcohol

The DSM-III-R lists a number of psychiatric disorders induced by alcohol. They include alcohol intoxication, idiosyncratic intoxication, withdrawal delirium, hallucinosis, amnestic disorder, and dementia associated with alcoholism. However, since most dually diagnosed patients use a variety of substances either at the same time or serially,[7-9] being able to identify psychotic symptoms seen in such an individual as being alcohol hallucinosis versus alcohol, marijuana, and/or cocaine idiosyncratic intoxication is problematic. In fact in many years of treating dually diagnosed patients I have only seen one clear case of alcohol hallucinosis admitted to our dually diagnosed program. On the other hand, our center treats hundreds of patients who have had temporary drug induced psychotic or paranoid symptoms after using a combination of cocaine, marijuana, alcohol, etc. Deciding as to which symptoms are caused by one drug or the other is of academic interest, however, it is rarely of much utility for the practicing clinician. Alcohol is the most available psychoactive substance of abuse to any patient of any diagnosis and thus is usually the most common drug found in dually diagnosed populations.[6-9] Its effects most often are seen in the context of (1) suicide attempts, (2) acting out behavior such as property destruction, threats to others, etc., and (3) alcohol use supplanting patients taking of medications, thus the schizophrenic or bipolar person decompensates into aggravated psychosis because of taking alcohol rather than taking prescribed medications such as neuroleptics or lithium.[8] Its effects are also seen when psychotic patients are admitted in an intoxicated condition and require treatment for alcohol withdrawal, confounding the diagnosis and treatment of the psychosis. These same patients may change their mind as to being in the hospital once they dry out.

A.2 Cocaine

Secondary to alcohol, marijuana and cocaine are the next most favored drugs in the dually diagnosed population seen at Harborview Medical Center. Cocaine and other potent stimulants have long been associated with the induction of psychotic and/or paranoid symptoms.[6] While it is currently uncommon to find a patient in 5-point restraints on our psychiatric unit with an aggressive drug induced psychosis due solely to alcohol, it is not so uncommon to find such patients with what appears to be an aggressive paranoid psychosis induced by cocaine or more often crack. It should be pointed out, however, that the bulk of such patients have also been using alcohol and often other drugs such as marijuana. Cocaine is encountered in dually diagnosed patients in the following manners:

(1) A brief but aggressive drug induced paranoid psychosis in a chronic polydrug abuser who has been using crack and other forms of cocaine along with alcohol. These patients are admitted on involuntary hold for being a danger to others or self and usually respond within hours or a day or two to unit structure and brief use of antipsychotic and/or benzodiazepine sedatives if needed.[10,11]

(2) The young chronic psychotic "street person" with either schizophrenia or unstable bipolar disorder who episodically abuses

cocaine, alcohol and marijuana. If such patients have the "good luck" to obtain or be able to afford the use of crack for a few days, they often decompensate with an aggravation of their baseline psychotic and/or mood symptoms and are admitted on involuntary treatment holds. In this kind of patient, two things are going on simultaneously: (a) the patient usually stops their baseline therapeutic psychiatric medications, and (b) the use of crack and alcohol aggravates their baseline psychiatric disorder.[9] There is some evidence that schizophrenics preferably abuse stimulants despite the apparent psychotomimetic effect.[7] This issue will be addressed in a later section under "self medication."

A.3 Marijuana

Numerous case reports and studies indicate that cannabis can cause psychotic symptoms that last from hours to even weeks.[10] While such case studies exist it is not our experience to see classical psychotic symptoms induced solely by cannabis. More likely cannabis use exacerbates psychotic symptoms or medication non-compliance in patients with major psychotic disorders such as schizophrenia, bipolar disorder, or other psychiatric conditions (see below). A few but pronounced cases of mania have been reported which followed heavy marijuana use. Dual diagnosis units see a small but regular number of patients admitted for depression and suicidal overdose who have been chronic marijuana users. These patients have often used marijuana for 5, 10 or 20 years and over a period of time have become less and less functional in their relationships, jobs and other activities.

A.4 Hallucinogens

As indicated by their very name, hallucinogens can induce psychotic symptoms. However, in recent years relatively few patients with acute psychoses due to hallucinogens have been admitted to our unit or reported in the literature. More commonly found, however, is the 23 or 24 year old psychotic patient with an early history of heavy marijuana and hallucinogen use throughout their teenage years. These patients are admitted with a schizophrenic-like presentation, however, often seem to have better social skills. Their symptoms may appear more "schizotypal," that is less florid and more likely "eccentric" or magical than a typical schizophrenic presentation. We usually give these kinds of patients a trial of carbamazepine in an attempt to block kindled hallucinogenic experiences.

A.5 Other Agents

While polydrug users will abuse virtually anything, the bulk of patients currently seem to use alcohol, marijuana, and cocaine, as has been found by others.[7-9] Few psychotic patients in our program use heroin on a regular basis. It appears that for patients with chronic unstable psychoses such as schizophrenia the complex behavior required to obtain money, obtain drugs, shoot up drugs, and repeat the cycle regularly is too difficult. More histories of heroin and/or other I.V. use are seen in non-psychotic patients. There is little evidence to show that use of opiates leads to psychotic symptoms.[10] We continue to hear from our colleagues at methadone clinics that there are patients who manifest psychotic symptoms once their methadone dose decreases to a certain point, however, we do not find these patients in our dually diagnosed programs. At times we have found psychotic patients abusing either prescribed or nonprescribed benzodiazepines. Recently benzodiazepines have been used increasingly in the managements of psychoses and mania,[11,12] and it is likely that we will see more cases of psychotic patients who have become dependent on benzodiazepines or who may abuse them by increasing doses, and/or combining them with alcohol or other drugs.

B. Non Drug Induced Psychoses in Which Substance Use May Contribute

As mentioned above, psychoses can and do exist separately from induced symptoms from drugs of abuse. Those psychiatric disorders most commonly seen in dually diagnosed programs include the following:

B.1 Schizophrenia

For discussion we will include schizophreniform disorder (a schizophrenic like condition lasting less than six months), schizoaffective disorder (schizophrenic like disease with prominent mood symptoms), and schizophrenia together in this section. Schizophrenia is characterized by (a) psychotic symptoms, (b) disturbance of functioning in work, social relationships, etc., (c) not being due to another mental disorder, and (d) continuous signs of the disturbance for at least six months. In schizophrenia "positive" psychotic symptoms are those such as auditory hallucinations and bizarre delusions, while negative symptoms are those which involve social withdrawal, flat affect, and passivity. Because of the relatively fragile mental status and instability of most schizophrenics, it is difficult to determine to what degree use, abuse or dependence on drugs destabilizes an already unstable condition. Schizophrenics are known to use alcohol, marijuana and cocaine frequently.[7,13-15] If such use leads to destabilization, increased psychotic symptoms, hospitalization, etc., then why do schizophrenics use drugs and alcohol? Is there some sort of "self medication?" In fact, the same questions can be asked of alcoholics who use alcohol. Why does an alcoholic who has increasing problems with health, job, and well-being continue to use alcohol despite adverse consequences? The answer to this question has been the development of the disease concept of addiction. That is, continued use despite adverse consequences is one of the key criteria for the diagnosis of both substance abuse and dependence. "Self medication" with alcohol and/or other drugs, despite adverse consequences is a key feature of alcoholics with alcoholism, as well as schizophrenics, manics, and others with alcoholism, or other drug dependency.

Research with dually diagnosed schizophrenics has found that drug and alcohol use varies a great deal. Despite some reports indicating schizophrenics prefer stimulants to alcohol or vice-a-versa,[7,13,14] none of the research findings are so robust as to be clinically helpful for any individual clinical case. Our experience suggests that schizophrenics tend to use the substances that are most readily available to them and thus environment and opportunity tend to determine use patterns. We also find it rare for patients who we determined to be "truly schizophrenic" that is, have clear evidence of established schizophrenia separate from any drug use or abuse, to be heavy users of any drug or alcohol regularly for long continuous periods of time. It appears that schizophrenics who attempt to use heavily and regularly tend to decompensate and end up in the hospital in which a forced period of abstinence occurs. Thus most of our dually diagnosed schizophrenic patients have drug and alcohol histories that are variable and episodic. Drugs and alcohol are most implicated in episodes of decompensation in which patients stop taking regularly prescribed medications, stop attending psychiatric or community mental health therapy, and end up admitted in a psychotic decompensated state.[9] Even in patients who do not decompensate so profoundly it is often the use of drugs or alcohol which leads to patients missing their appointments or other responsibilities.

Because a significant part of the schizophrenic picture is abnormal and/or bizarre communication, special considerations regarding their chemical dependency treatment will need to be addressed.[16-19] Also, since most schizophrenics will be maintained on a psychiatric medication, special issues regarding the use of medications need also to be addressed (see below).

B.2 Mania

Core features of mania are poor impulse control and over involvement in many kinds of problematic behaviors including substance abuse, spending, and sex. Therefore, with manics more than other diagnoses the question is asked, "Is the substance abuse just a 'symptom' of mania, or is it really a separate problem?" Addressing this question is important since its answer may guide clinicians to focus on different interventions. Mania also seems to be the most usual diagnosis in which the concept of "self medication" is employed. "Self medication" for manics implies that they medicate their hyperactive symptoms with a sedative such as alcohol. Since clinicians medicate manics in the hospital with major tranquilizers and benzodiazepine sedatives, this concept makes sense to them. But does this conceptualization help or hinder treatment? Manics may be extremely psychotic at times, however, unlike most schizophrenics, they may have long periods with essentially normal mental status. This allows most manics (once stabilized) to participate in regular chemical dependency treatment services.

B.3 Depression

While depression combined with substance use is among the most common "dual diagnoses" overall,[5] psychotic depression combined with active substance use appears infrequently. In the Harborview program we have seen several patients with histories of chemical dependency who have later developed psychotic depressions but very few patients diagnosed with psychotic depression who have concurrent substance abuse or dependence.

B.4 Brief Reactive Psychosis

Brief reactive psychosis is a psychosis induced by a well defined severe stress causing a temporary psychosis whose content usually involves some aspect of the stress. Brief reactive psychosis is a relatively rare phenomenon and we see little of it in our dual diagnosis program.

B.5 Dissociative Disorders

Dissociative disorders and PTSD have received increasing attention in the last 10 to 15 years.[20] Many of the more severe dissociative conditions are found in persons who have been abused as children,[10,21] and among multiproblem inner city patients significant histories of sexual and physical abuse as children exist.[21] Dissociative disorders may mimic active psychosis in certain patients.[20] Patients who complain of "voices" or thoughts of control who otherwise have nearly normal mental status examinations and who were abused as children are likely candidates for having dissociative disorders versus schizophrenia or other kinds of psychoses. Dissociative patients do not respond to neuroleptics very well and may have many other "personality" kinds of presentations such as borderline personality disorder.[20]

B.6 Organic Brain Damage

Organic brain damage may occur as a result of trauma, drug or alcohol ingestion, or other medical disorder. Frequently organic brain damaged patients have difficulties with cognition and impulse control thus making rational decisions about substance use difficult. The psychotic symptoms in such a patient will often be disorganized and confused resembling more of a delirium than a schizophrenic or manic picture. Thus, such a patient may appear to be a case of extreme toxicity which is resistant to treatment.[6]

C. Prevalence of Combined Psychosis and Substance Disorders

National prevalence statistics such as those developed by the ECA (Epidemiologic Catchment Area program) study indicate that schizophrenics have an increased use and prevalence of alcohol and drug disorders.[5] Other data indicate that those persons without a formal mental disorder who use alcohol, cocaine, or marijuana on a regular basis have an increased risk for psychotic experiences when screened for them.[10] Studies which have looked at young adult chronic psychotic patients in urban areas find substance abuse in over 50% of the cases.[1,7,8,22] On the other hand, Rounsaville and colleagues found almost no cases of schizophrenia in their careful study of treatment-seeking cocaine abusers.[23] Does this mean that psychotic cocaine abusers don't seek treatment? Probably not; more likely it means that certain kinds of patients are found in certain kinds of places. Screening and referral programs for cocaine treatment facilities most likely screen out those patients with bizarre, disruptive or clearly inappropriate behaviors. On the other hand, substance using psychotic patients who repeatedly fail both inpatient and outpatient therapies are likely to be found in the urban case managed kinds of populations such as those reported in the psychiatric "young adult chronic populations."[1,8,9,14,16,17] Thus, different treatment sites select for different kinds of patients and prevalence studies will likely reveal upfront selection processes more than they particularly reveal the nature of a larger population. Knowing the prevalence and nature of problems in the particular clinic or population in which one practices is what matters.

D. Self Medication Hypothesis

As referenced above, there appears to be an inherent conflict in two sets of research reports. One set of reports indicates that schizophrenics increasingly abuse alcohol, cocaine, marijuana and other drugs, especially stimulants, over the general population.[6,9,22] Another set of reports indicates that schizophrenics who take psychoactive drugs, especially stimulants, get worse.[13-15] Why then would schizophrenics "self medicate" with drugs such as amphetamines or cocaine if research indicates their psychotic symptoms will likely get worse? There are several theories which might be developed:

(1) Schizophrenics or other psychotics don't always get worse, sometimes they may feel more relaxed, euphoric, and/or social, just as many normals do, when taking recreational drugs or other substances. Even though their psychotic symptoms may get worse, the positive euphoriant or relaxant properties of the substance may be powerful enough to keep the person using despite negative psychotic consequences.[3,14]

(2) Many psychotic patients are drug or alcohol dependent. A key feature of psychoactive substance dependence is continued use despite adverse consequences. As pointed out above, alcoholics continue to drink alcohol despite significantly negative social, family, health and job consequences. In fact, the most clear case of self medication is the alcoholic. The alcoholic self medicates with alcohol and alcoholism is a disorder of alcohol self medication, despite adverse consequences.

(3) A certain number of psychotics, those who are on antipsychotic medication, use drugs or alcohol to medicate the side effects of psychiatric medications. While there is no clear documentation for this type of use with cocaine, alcohol or marijuana, there is evidence that nicotine reverses some of the unpleasant side effects of neuroleptics.[24] Flat affect, anhedonia, and low energy are common side effects of neuroleptic medications, and stimulants may temporarily reduce these symptoms. Biologically, neuroleptics block dopamine and stimulants increase it. It might be that schizophrenics are attempting to rebalance a neuroleptic blocked dopamine system.

Probably the best study related to "self medication" was done by Bernadt and Murray in the United Kingdom.[25] Patients were diagnosed according to the Research Diagnostic Criteria, and increase or decrease in alcohol use in the month prior to admission was carefully studied. The only group of patients who increased alcohol use in a significant fashion in the month prior to admission were those with a diagnosis of alcoholism. Other disorders such as bipolar manic, depression, anxiety, and schizophrenia were found to have a different pattern: that is, the bulk of patients didn't change their drinking and about as many decreased their use of alcohol as increased their alcohol prior to admission. Thus, if the 20% of manics who increased their drinking prior to admission are called "self medicators" should the 25% of manics who decreased their drinking prior to admission as their mania was developing be called "anti-self medicators" and should the ones who did not change their use of substances be called "non-self medicators?" What characterizes the "self medicators" from the "anti-self medicators" and/or the "non-self medicators?" It appears from both Bernadt's work[25] and others,[26] that those patients who drink more as they are getting worse (isn't this drinking despite adverse consequences?) are those who qualify as having a substance use disorder. At this point, things appear to be getting circular and one wonders what purpose the "self medication" hypothesis might serve, other than to rationalize (by the clinician and/or patient) a substance use condition without recognizing it as a problem needing specific addiction interventions.

Clinicians uncomfortable with substance intervention or treatment may prefer to believe that substance use disorders will disappear if they treat the "core" condition of mania, schizophrenia or other more comfortable psychiatric diagnosis. This is not our experience, nor that of multiple other programs[2-5,16-19] that have found that specific interventions for both psychiatric and addiction disorder must be designed. Substance interventions developed by such programs, usually mimic those which have been developed within the addiction treatment field.

II. TREATMENT

Once diagnosis has been clarified using some of the principles outlined above, appropriate treatment should match the appropriate condition. Using the low/high severity model outlined above to recharacterize the patient as the acute condition resolves (in order to plan for longer term treatment needs) is important. For example, patients with drug induced psychoses which have completely resolved need to be out of the psychiatric system and into the addiction treatment system. Patients with longer term psychotic disorders such as schizophrenia will likely need a combination of case management, day treatment, and medications, as well as focus on their substance use disorder depending on whether it is abuse or dependence. Interventions for episodic use or abuse can be educationally oriented and provided within the context of typical psychiatric care. However, if dependence is present, more time and effort focusing on the substance disorder and involvement with addiction treatment resources will be needed. A more detailed description of this process is provided elsewhere.[4] Space limitations prevent a conclusive review of all of the elements needed for treatment of the psychotic dual diagnosed patient. However, readers are referred to several excellent sources on the following topics: inpatient dual diagnosis units,[3,4,16-19] use of 12-steps (Alcoholics Anonymous,[16,17]) psychiatric versus addiction concepts,[3,4,16,18] acute, subacute, and longer term psychiatric management.

Since psychiatric medications play such a central role in the treatment of psychoses, a special section on psychiatric medications is provided.

A. Psychiatric Medications in the Psychotic Dually Diagnosed Patient

The following medications will be discussed in this section:

1. Antipsychotic
2. Antimanic
3. Antianxiety/sedative agents
4. Antidepressants
5. Anticholinergics

Detailed pharmacological description of each agent can be found in standard psychopharmacological texts. For the purpose of this work each class of medications will be discussed around three particular relevant issues for dual diagnosis patients:

1. What is the abuse potential of the medication.
2. What characteristics of the medication may help sobriety or recovery.
3. What characteristics of the medication may hinder sobriety or recovery.

A.1 Antipsychotics

Abuse Potential–Though millions of doses of antipsychotics have been given, there are virtually no substance abuse reports for the antipsychotics. In fact, the main problem with antipsychotics is getting patients (especially dually diagnosed) who need them to take them.[9]

Help Recovery–Antipsychotics can help recovery by allowing those patients who need them to participate in treatment, AA meetings or other recovery resources. There is some evidence that the dopamine blocking characteristics of antipsychotics interfere with the euphoric effect of stimulants such as cocaine which work through dopamine transmission.[27]

Hinder Recovery–Antipsychotics cause dysphoria and other unpleasant side effects in both psychotic and nonpsychotic individuals. As stated above, the main obstacle in using antipsychotics is getting patients to take them in the first place. Because they often cause unpleasant side effects, patients may use drugs or alcohol in an attempt to reverse the dysphoria or akathesia that they may cause.[13,14] Thus, while helping a patient with psychosis, the antipsychotic medications may cause so many side effects that the patient turns to drugs or alcohol in an attempt to feel better. For this and other reasons using antipsychotics for acute management of suspected drug induced psychoses may backfire. Since most antipsychotics stay in the system for several days to weeks following acute dosages, even if a drug induced psychosis responds to their use, their carryover effect may push the patient into further drug use. And if not further drug use, side effects may alienate patients from the therapist or clinic. Therefore, acute use of benzodiazepines as first line medications (see below), may be preferable.

A.2 Antimanic Agents

Abuse Potential–There are several classes of antimanic medications, chiefly (1) lithium, (2) anticonvulsants, and (3) benzodiazepines. We will discuss benzodiazepines below under that section. Neither lithium nor anticonvulsants have significant abuse potential. Again, though less so than with antipsychotics, the main problem with both sets of agents is getting patients who need them to take them.

Help Recovery–Antimanic agents should help recovery by allowing a manic patient to function more normally and participate in recovery. An untreated manic cannot participate in either psychiatric or chemical dependency recovery. Some years ago it was thought that lithium might help alcoholics to decrease their use of alcohol and thus recover more effectively; however, newer research has not corroborated this.[28] Anti-convulsant agents such as carbamazepine and sodium valproate, have become increasingly used in treating bipolar disorder. They help with recovery in the same way that lithium does by stabilizing the patient's mental status enough so that they may participate in both psychiatric and chemical dependency treatment. Both carbamazepine and valproate have been found to be effective in alcohol and benzodiazepine withdrawal treatments such that a manic who is also in alcohol withdrawal can be treated safely with one agent, i.e., carbamazepine.[29,30] There have also been preliminary reports that cocaine users use less cocaine when taking carbamazepine.[31]

Hinder Recovery–Lithium's main side effects include tremor, nausea and skin irritations. If patients are in the therapeutic window, none of these side effects are usually prominent enough to hinder substance recovery and many patients participate fully in chemical recovery while taking lithium. Carbamazepine's main side effects are nausea and sedation. If patients adapt to these effects over the first week or two, usually no further problem exists and they can participate fully. Valproate has fewer side effects than carbamazepine and thus is usually no problem. However, certain patients may be intolerant of one or another medication and bad medication side effects with any agent may lead to medication noncompliance and/or use of substances.

A.3 Antianxiety/Sedatives

The main agents in current use are the benzodiazepines. Benzodiazepines have been used increasingly in the management of acute psychosis, mania,[11,12] and even antipsychotic side effects. This is because they are fast, predictable and are absorbed readily IM, IV or PO. A variety of agents exists such that those with different half lives can be used according to patient's clinical needs.

Abuse Potential–Benzodiazepines vary a great deal in terms of their psychoactivity and abuse/dependence potential.[32] Shorter acting more highly lipid soluble agents appear to be more psychoactive and are rated as higher on the abuse potential. Older longer-acting agents such as chlordiazepoxide and clonazepam apparently have little abuse potential although it does exist.[33]

Help Recovery–Benzodiazepines are also the most usual treatment for alcohol and other sedative withdrawal. Since they are first line drugs for both behavioral and withdrawal treatment, they are often a good choice in the acute dual diagnosis patient, since many come in with both psychotic agitation and alcohol withdrawal at the same time. However, since they may induce dependence, especially over time, we recommend only acute and not longer term use of benzodiazepines.

Hinder Recovery–Benzodiazepine dependence is most commonly found in patients addicted to other drugs of abuse (i.e., dually diagnosed patients); therefore, other methods for longer term treatment should be employed. Benzodiazepines might theoretically help recovery by stabilizing the mental condition sufferer thus allowing the patient to participate more fully in recovery treatment. However, since tolerance and dependence develops more rapidly to benzodiazepines in patients with alcoholic histories, more and more of the benzodiazepine is usually needed in order to attain the same affect. This causes dose escalation and often alcohol use. In addition, pharmacological dependence has been shown to develop in virtually all users, beyond a few weeks.[32] Pharmocologic dependence produces anxiety during medication withdrawal, thus complicating both the diagnosis of anxiety as well as its appropriate treatment in such patients.

A.4 Antidepressants

Abuse Potential–There are a wide variety of antidepressants on the market ranging from tricyclics to newer non-cyclic agents. While there are more case reports indicating "abuse" of antidepressants than antipsychotics or antimanic medications, this at most represents a rare finding. None of the currently available antidepressants on the market pharmacologically mimic the activities of the major drugs of abuse. The antidepressant which is closest in pharmacological structure is buproprion. The buproprion molecule is amphetamine like in structure and different clinicians have used the similarity for two different hypothetical stands: (1) Buproprion should be given to patients with a history of stimulant abuse since they have already "self selected" for this genre of medication. (2) Buproprion should not be given to patients with substance abuse histories since they may abuse it. No clear evidence exists to support either of these hypothetical stands and clinicians are recommended to follow developing research evidence around these issues.

Help Recovery–The elegant work of Dixon et al.[13] suggests that while schizophrenics get more psychotic with substance use, they claim to get relief from their anhedonia, depression, and other negative symptoms by this same substance use. But do antidepressants help nonspecific dysphoric symptoms in recovering substance abusers? In preliminary studies antidepressants have been shown to favorable effect the treatment for cocaine[33] and nicotine addiction,[34] however, it is unclear as to whether this is an "antidepressant" or other pharmacological effect.

Hinder Recovery–While antidepressants should clearly be considered for a "recovering" patient who has a major depression, the use of antidepressants in a psychotic or previously psychotic individual is of more concern. Antidepressants may cause schizophrenics to experience more psychotic symptoms, and may switch some bipolar depressed patients into mania.

A.5 Anticholinergic Agents

Abuse Potential–Anticholinergic agents are used to combat many of the side effects of neuroleptics. A significant number of reports of abuse by patients, as well as the selling of anticholinergics by patients to addicts exists.[36] It appears that addicts, especially heroin addicts, may get a buzz by taking anticholinergic agents on top of their injected heroin.

Help Recovery–Anticholinergic agents could indeed help recovery by blocking some of the unpleasant side effects from antipsychotic patients. If a schizophrenic is taking an antipsychotic and experiencing severe side effects, they may turn to drugs or alcohol for temporary relief. Appropriate use of an anticholinergic agent may make the patient comfortable enough that they can better take part in both psychiatric and/or substance abuse recovery treatment. There is no known anti-addiction property of anticholinergic drugs.

Hinder Recovery–As mentioned above, anticholinergics have a certain but small abuse potential. Thus, they may hinder recovery by promoting abuse of the agents themselves in a certain number of patients. Also, patients may be overmedicated with anticholinergic medications thus causing dry mouth, inability to focus vision on near objects and constipation. It is likely that the more uncomfortable a patient is, the more probable they are to relapse to drug use. Likewise they would be less likely to be able to participate in either substance or psychiatric recovery programs.

A.6 General Medication Issues

As discussed above, all of the medications may help and/or hinder recovery, and some have abuse potential. Beyond these properties is the issue of whether a patient taking any medication whatsoever can participate in "recovery." While less commonly encountered now than in the past, patients may still receive antimedication messages within the recovering community. AA World Services prints a pamphlet supporting the use of nonaddicting psychiatric medications such as antidepressants, lithium and antipsychotics for those patients who need them and who are under a doctor's supervision.[37] Patients should be told about potential antimedication bias and should be rehearsed on how to respond if the issue comes up. A separate issue is that psychiatrists and other mental health workers may focus more on medication issues than addiction recovery thus giving the patient the message that what counts is taking pills rather than getting sober. This type of response may encourage denial that addiction problems exist.

A reasonable guideline to decrease such denial is that clinicians who treat dual diagnosis patients with medications should spend at least as much time talking to them about addiction treatment and recovery as they do about medication effects or side effects.

REFERENCES

1. Lehman AF, Myers CP, Corty E. Assessment and classification of patients with psychiatric and substance abuse syndromes. Hospital and Community Psychiatry 1989; 40(10):1037-1040.

2. Shuckit M. Clinical implications of primary diagnostic groups among alcoholics. Arch General Psychiatry 1985; 42:1043-1049.

3. Wallen M, Weiner H. The dually diagnosed patient in an inpatient chemical dependency treatment program. Alcoholism Treatment Quarterly 1988; 5(1/2): 197-218.

4. Ries RK, Miller NS. Dual diagnosis: Concept, diagnosis, and treatment. In: Dunner DL, ed. Current Psychiatric Therapy. Philadelphia: W.B. Saunders Co.: In Press.

5. Reiger DA, Farmer ME, Rae DS, Locke BZ, Keith SJ, Judd LL, Goodwin FK. Comorbidity of mental disorders with alcohol and other drug abuse. JAMA 1990; 264(19):3511-2518.

6. Mirin SM, Weiss RD. Substance abuse and mental illness. In: Frances RJ, Miller S, ed. Clinical Textbook of Addictive Disorders. New York: The Guilford Press, 1991:282-286.

7. Schneier FR, Siris SG. A review of psychoactive use and abuse in schizophrenia: Patterns of drug choice. Journal of Nervous & Mental Disease 1987; 175(11):641-652.

8. Galanter M, Castaneda R, Ferman J. Substance abuse among general psychiatric patients. Hospital & Community Psychiatry 1989; 40(10):1041-1045.

9. Drake RE, Wallach MA. Substance abuse among the chronic mentally ill. Hospital and Community Psychiatry 1989; 40(10):1041-1045.

10. Tien AY, Anthony JC. Epidemiological analysis of alcohol and drug use as risk factors for psychotic experiences. The Journal of Nervous & Mental Disease 1990; 178(8):473-480.

11. Wolkowitz OM, Pickar D. Benzodiazepines in the treatment of schizophrenia: A review and reappraisal. American Journal of Psychiatry 1991; 148(6): 714-726.

12. Cohen S, Khan A, Johnson S. Pharmacological management of manic psychosis in an unlocked setting. Journal Clinical Psychopharmacology 1987; 7(4): 261-264.

13. Dixon L, Haas G. Weiden P, Sweeney J, Frances A. Acute effects of drug abuse in schizophrenic patients: Clinical observations and patients' self-reports. Schizophrenia Bulletin 1990; 16(1):69-79.

14. Castaneda R, Galanter M, Franco H. Self-medication among addicts with primary psychiatric disorders. Comprehensive Psychiatry 1989; 30(1):80-83.

15. Brady K, Anton R, Ballenger JC, Lydiard RB, Adinoff B, Selander J. Cocaine abuse among schizophrenic patients. American Journal of Psychiatry 1990; 147(9):1164-1167.

16. Minkoff K. An integrated treatment model for dual diagnosis of psychosis and addiction. Hospital & Community Psychiatry 1989; 40(10):1031-1036.

17. Osher FC, Kofoed LL. Treatment of patients with psychiatric and psychoactive substance abuse disorders. Hospital & Community Psychiatry 1989; 40(10):1025-1030.

18. Evans K, Sullivan JM. Dual Diagnosis: Counseling the mentally ill substance abuser. New York: The Guilford Press, 1990.

19. O'Connell DF. Managing the dually diagnosed patient. In: O'Connell DF, ed. Current issues and clinical approaches. New York: The Haworth Press, 1990.

20. Kluft RP. First-rank symptoms as a diagnostic clue to multiple personality disorder. American Journal of Psychiatry 1987; 144(3):293-298.

21. Brown GR, Anderson B. Psychiatric morbidity in adult inpatients with childhood histories of sexual and physical abuse. American Journal of Psychiatry 1991; 148(1):55-61.

22. Salloum IM, Moss HB, Daley DC. Substance Abuse and Schizophrenia: Impediments to optimal care. American Journal of Drug & Alcohol Abuse 1991; 17(3):321-336.

23. Rounsaville BJ, Anton SF, Carroll K, Budde D, Prusoff BA, Gawin F. Psychiatric diagnoses of treatment-seeking cocaine abusers. Arch General Psychiatry 1991; 48:43-51.

24. Decina P, Caracci G, Sandik R, Berman W, Mukherjee S, Scapicchio P. Cigarette smoking and neuroleptic-induced parkinsonism. Society of Biological Psychiatry 1990; 28:502-508.

25. Bernadt MW, Murray RM. Psychiatric disorder, drinking and alcoholism: What are the links? British Journal of Psychiatry 1986; 148:393-400.

26. Miller NS. Drug and alcohol addiction as a disease. In: Miller NS ed. Comprehensive handbook of drug and alcohol addiction. New York: Marcel Dekker, Inc., 1991:295-309.

27. Gawin FH, Allen D, Humblestone B. Outpatient treatment of 'crack' cocaine smoking with flupenthixol decanoate. Arch Gen Psychiatry 1989; 46: 322-325.

28. Clark DC, Fawcett J. Does lithium carbonate therapy for alcoholism deter relapse drinking? In: Galanter M, Ed. Recent developments in alcoholism: Volume 7 Treatment Research. New York: Plenum Press, 1989:315-328.

29. Ries RK, Cullison S, Horn R, Ward N. Benzodiazepine withdrawal: Clinician's ratings of carbamazepine treatment versus traditional taper methods. Journal of Psychoactive Drugs 1991; 23(1):73-76.

30. Malcolm R, Ballenger JC, Sturgis ET, Anton R. Double-blind controlled trial comparing carbamazepine to oxazepam treatment of alcohol withdrawal. American Journal of Psychiatry 1989; 146:617-621.

31. Halikas J, Kemp K, Kuhn K, Carlson G, Crea F. Carbamazepine for cocaine addiction? Lancet 1989; 1(8638):623-624.

32. Griffiths RR, Wolf B. Relative abuse liability of different benzodiazepines in drug abusers. Journal of Clinical Psychopharmacology 1990; 10(4):237-243.

33. Baron DH, Sands BF, Ciraulo D, Shader RI. The diagnosis and treatment of panic disorder in alcoholics: Three cases. American Journal of Drug and Alcohol Abuse 1990; 16(3&4):287-295.

34. Gawin FH, Fleber HD, Byck R, et al. Desipramine facilitation of initial cocaine abstinence. Arch General Psychiatry 1989; 46:117-121.

35. Murphy JK, Edwards NB, Downs AD, Ackerman BJ, Rosenthal TL. Effects of doxepin on withdrawal symptoms in smoking cessation. American Journal of Psychiatry 1990: 147(10):1353-1357.

36. Dilsaver SC. Antimuscarinic agents as substances of abuse: A review. Journal of Clinical Psychopharmacology 1988; 8(1):14-22.

37. Alcoholics Anonymous World Services, Inc. The AA Member-Medications and Other Drugs, New York, 1984.

Outpatient vs. Inpatient Treatment for the Chronically Mentally Ill with Substance Use Disorders

Lial Kofoed, MD, MS

SUMMARY. Treatment decisions about complex patients with both substance use disorders and chronic mental illness cannot be reduced to an inpatient vs. outpatient dichotomy. Treatment progresses through a series of stages, in each of which we must make decisions about treatment settings and approaches. I discuss treatment decisions within the framework of a staged treatment model, reviewing decisions to be made during stabilization, engagement, persuasion, active (or primary) treatment, and relapse prevention (or aftercare).

Treatment decisions about our multidiagnosis, multiproblem chronic patients cannot be reduced to simple inpatient vs. outpatient decisions. There are distinct phases of treatment, and resources and

Lial Kofoed is Research Director and Professor, Department of Psychiatry, University of South Dakota School of Medicine, and Staff Psychiatrist at the VA Medical Center in Sioux Falls, SD.

Correspondence and reprint requests should be addressed to Dr. Lial Kofoed, Psychiatry Service (116 A), Royal C. Johnson VAMC, P.O. Box 5046, Sioux Falls, SD 57117.

[Haworth co-indexing entry note]: "Outpatient vs. Inpatient Treatment for the Chronically Mentally Ill with Substance Use Disorders." Kofoed, Lial. Co-published simultaneously in *Journal of Addictive Diseases,* (The Haworth Press, Inc.) Vol. 12, No. 3, 1993, pp. 123-137; and: *Comorbidity of Addictive and Psychiatric Disorders* (Ed: Norman S. Miller, and Barry Stimmel) The Haworth Press, Inc., 1993, pp. 123-137. Multiple copies of this article/chapter may be purchased from The Haworth Document Delivery Center. Call 1-800-3-HAWORTH (1-800-342-9678) between 9:00 - 5:00(EST) and ask for DOCUMENT DELIVERY CENTER.

settings required for effective treatment will vary as differing patients progress through these stages. Furthermore, there are some times choices between differing outpatient or distinct inpatient treatments. Choosing the most effective treatment approach in each stage requires familiarity with the clinical literature, common sense, and a good touch of the art of medicine. The diagnoses, predominant symptoms, and social and cultural factors unique to each patient will affect their responses to differing treatments. Thus in this chapter I will discuss treatment decisions in terms of the stages of treatment and the needs common to patients in each stage. Drawing on a sequential treatment model, I will overview factors important in selection of appropriate treatment settings, discuss specific treatment components, and review and apply pertinent clinical literature. The discussion will emphasize treatment choices for patients with both chronic mental illness and a substance use disorder.

WHO NEEDS DUAL DIAGNOSIS TREATMENT?

We often think of this population as defined by diagnoses. However McLellan and colleagues[1] have demonstrated that the variable most predictive of poor substance abuse treatment outcome in a variety of primary substance abuse treatment programs is overall severity of psychiatric symptoms. Patients with severe psychiatric symptoms apparently require specialized treatment regardless of the diagnosis underlying the symptoms. Perhaps most difficult are patients with Axis I diagnoses that in themselves follow a chronic course (i.e., schizophrenia, schizo-affective disorder, bipolar disorder, or the severe anxiety disorders). Diagnosis is necessary to develop effective differential treatment for psychiatric symptoms, but does not lead automatically to all treatment planning decisions. Kofoed[2] has provided a review of assessment dimensions and instruments pertinent to treatment planning for dual diagnosis patients.

TREATMENT STAGES

Osher and Kofoed[3] have suggested that patients entering treatment "are likely to be in different phases of illness and recovery, given the chronic relapsing course of . . . (the) . . . disorders, the variation in individuals' abilities to form treatment relationships, and differences in previous exposure to treatment" (p. 1026). Treatment must progress through these phases. I will discuss inpatient and outpatient resources and differential treatment planning for sequential treatment stages beginning with *stabilization* (including intoxication and detoxification), progressing through *engagement, persuasion, active (or primary) treatment,* and *relapse prevention (or aftercare),* and will review the potential of substance abuse specific pharmacologic agents to enhance the efficacy of treatment decisions.

STABILIZATION

Certain medical and psychiatric needs demand immediate attention in treatment planning. The presence of intoxication, risk of a serious withdrawal syndrome, or emergent psychiatric and behavioral risk demands our clinical attention. Decisions about treatment setting are critical in safely managing patients during stabilization.

Intoxication

The intoxicated dual diagnosis patient often presents unpleasant clinical dilemmas. Intoxication itself is a difficult, erratic state with exaggerated presentation of baseline symptoms. Unfortunately intoxication is also a period of increased risk of acting out or destructive behavior. While not always considered, intoxication is also a period of increased risk for victimization; many victims of assault or homicide are intoxicated when victimized.

Since intoxication with most drugs, including alcohol, impairs abstract cognitive functioning and ability to acquire new information, attempts at therapy during intoxication are not of much value (I don't usually do psychotherapy with anesthetized patients, either!). Thus the major issue becomes risk assessment and management. Patients often report suicidal or assaultive ideation during intoxication; assessment of this risk and the risk of victimization may determine the need for a controlled setting. This need presents a dilemma for those working with dual diagnosis patients because many community resources are unwilling to accept patients "tainted" with a psychiatric label. Although non-medical detoxification resources are some times willing to accept such patients, more commonly brief police custody (protective custody) must be employed, with patients returned to the clinical setting for further evaluation of risk when less intoxicated. Often the inpatient psychiatry ward becomes the only resource accessible to such patients, particularly if intoxication has exaggerated psychiatric symptoms and erratic behaviors. Pinsker[4] suggests reasonable goals when intoxicated dual diagnosis patients must be admitted to general psychiatry units for management. Providing structure and behavioral control, rapidly treating worsened psychiatric symptoms, monitoring detoxification, and working to engage and persuade the patient to accept the necessary multi-focused ongoing rehabilitative treatment are all helpful and manageable on general psychiatry units.

Detoxification

Discussion of managing intoxication has already led naturally to discussion of detoxification. This rather odd term implies removal of the effects of the intoxicant, but has come to include management of withdrawal or abstinence phenomena. As a consequence of medical training physicians think of detoxification primarily in terms of pharmacologic withdrawal. However in many primary substance abusers non-medical approaches (often grouped together as "social detox") appear safe and effective.[5] Dual diagnosis patients unfortunately may present disruptive symptoms that are poorly tolerated by social detox programs; conversely their need for pharmacologic treatment of withdrawal is probably no higher than that of primary alcoholics. During pre-admission drug or alcohol abuse patients often become non-compliant with prescribed medication,[6] so that they require stabilization of psychiatric symptoms concurrently with detoxification.[7]

Assessment of the need for hospitalization can be aided by an assessment of the risk of a severe abstinence syndrome. In the case of alcohol use, administering a breathalyzer and concurrently rating alcohol withdrawal symptoms may be helpful. Patients who show marked tachycardia, systolic hypertension, hyper-reflexia, or fine tremor (differentiation from a neuroleptic-induced Parkinsonian tremor must be made) in the face of a non-zero BAC are at risk of significant abstinence symptoms. Patients with a history of severe withdrawal reactions are also at increased risk. Estimating withdrawal risk from patient accounts of consumption is not very useful.

In the absence of serious withdrawal risk, assessment of likely compliance with outpatient treatment must be made, and the patient's need for acute psychiatric symptom control assessed. In the presence of an established treatment relationship and a psychiatric status that permits reliable follow-up, detoxification and stabilization of psychiatric symptoms may often be managed on an outpatient basis.

Patient self-reports of motivation may prove useful in assessing the probability that they will follow-up appropriately with needed treatment. Ries et al.[8] showed that patient self-reports of motivation for abstinence early in treatment were significantly predictive of abstinence at short-term follow-up. This promising lead deserves further study in patients in varying stages of treatment.

ENGAGEMENT

Osher and Kofoed[3] define engagement as "convincing patients that the mental health agency . . . has something to offer them" (p. 1026). This phase may incorporate detoxification, since such help is a concrete offering. The process of engagement does not require an inpatient vs. outpatient decision; however legitimate offerings of help must be made in either setting for treatment to progress. Helpful enticements include effective relief from distressing symptoms, material help such as clothing, food, or housing assistance, or for capable patients access to recreation, socialization, or vocational rehabilitation.[3] Some patients will not accept inpatient treatment; isolated or homeless patients may require assertive outreach and concrete help, including support during crises.[9] Other patients may see the offer of admission as a great relief and an extremely valuable help. This in itself is a legitimate indication for admission, which can then proceed to focus on persuasion and treatment planning.

Engagement is not simply a matter of carrots; sticks may be applied simultaneously. Denial is a very real phenomenon even in the most impaired dual diagnosis patients. The combination of denial, disorganization, and loss of hope prevents some patients from responding to even the most positive and immediate offers of help. In such circumstances clinicians must welcome any opportunities for coercion. When patients experience legal difficulties, for instance, recommending strategies such as deferred sentencing with required treatment may produce involvement that would otherwise not occur. In some states options for outpatient commitment exist, and may be particularly applicable to this difficult population. The simultaneous offer of helpful services will help patients move from coerced to voluntary treatment involvement.

PERSUASION

Persuasion entails convincing patients to accept ongoing rehabilitative treatment. Dual diagnosis patients must come to accept ongoing help for both their psychiatric and substance use disorders. This requires that they begin to develop an understanding of the consequences and interplay of their dual illnesses, and of their inability to retain reliable control of their illnesses in the absence of treatment. The psychological goal of persuasion is to move patients from the external motivations (enticement and coercion) of the engagement stage to the internal motivation required for successful recovery.

I have come to emphasize persuasion as a distinct phase of treatment because there is evidence that a variety of pre-treatment interventions may make a difference in treatment acceptance rates both in primary substance abusers[10,11] and in dual diagnosis patients.[12] This phase is both especially difficult and especially important in dual diagnosis patients for several reasons. They are often unemployed so are not identified by Employee Assistance Programs, may not drive and hence won't receive DWIs, and even if arrested for an intoxication related offense may be excused by virtue of obvious mental illness. Thus they tend to escape the usual social and legal pressures which lead primary substance abusers into treatment. In the absence of these social and legal mechanisms, persuasive efforts by treating clinicians become even more important.

Pretreatment outpatient interventions in primary substance abusers successfully utilize both individual and group approaches.[10,11]

Persuasion can be undertaken with dual diagnosis outpatients under certain conditions. Psychiatric symptoms must be well enough controlled that patients can understand content and keep follow-up appointments. Often such patients will already be engaged in outpatient psychiatric treatment, having been referred because of refractory substance abuse. Specific data about outpatient persuasion of dual diagnosis patients is not available. Kofoed et al.[13] provide anecdotal data suggesting that individual outpatient persuasive efforts may be productive. Hellerstein and Meehan[14] incorporated elements of engagement and persuasion into outpatient group treatment, and reported success in retaining patients in the treatment group.

Inpatient persuasion may be particularly effective for several reasons. Inpatients experience forced sobriety, have psychiatric symptoms relatively well controlled, and by virtue of their inpatient status must admit things have gone wrong. Denial is thus more difficult to maintain, and patients may be particularly accessible to persuasion. Inpatient persuasion may also provide opportunities for productive peer interactions. Kofoed and Keys[12] described and provided data on an inpatient persuasion group which met only twice a week, yet demonstrated modest effectiveness in improving the percentage of patients accepting ongoing treatment which included a substance abuse focus.

Regardless of the setting of persuasive treatment, the underlying principles are similar. In order for patients to internalize motivation for ongoing treatment focused on stability and sobriety, they must develop both a conceptual understanding of and an emotional commitment to these goals. Clinicians must be willing to present the diagnoses with clarity and certainty. I believe the most useful conceptualization of the substance use disorders is that they are exemplified by a lesion of *control*.[15] Patients with these disorders do not have *reliable* control. They sometimes consume intoxicants when they don't mean to, or in excess of what they intend, or to the point of adverse consequences. The concept of unreliable control, as contrasted to complete loss of control, is critical. Even the most severely affected patients will experience brief periods when they feel in control. This conceptualization is also critical to help patients understand the reasons for complete abstinence. I often compare attempts at controlled use to throwing matches on a pile of rags in the attic. Any given match may not ignite the rags, but all are a risk, and if the rags ignite the entire house burns down.

The difficulty of reliably controlling, or even reliably self-identifying, psychiatric symptoms can be similarly discussed.[7] Discussion must be individualized to the patient's own experience of symptoms, consequences, and treatments.

While these concepts can be presented didactically, it's most effective to present them in the context of an individual or group session where examples of unreliable control have spontaneously come up. Linkage of the concepts to personal experience in this immediate fashion has maximum intellectual and emotional impact.

Many experienced clinicians believe that peer group discussion can be critical in helping patients attain both the conceptual and emotional goals of persuasion. Denial and defensiveness are reduced in peer interactions. There is a natural credibility and a sharing of culture, language, and experience not always available in interactions with professionals. Recovering counselors with training in the needs of psychiatrically ill substance abusers may provide an effective blend of professionalism and credibility. For these same reasons Twelve Step recovery groups may be of great help to patients during this stage, if the particular group attended is tolerant of psychiatric symptoms and the possible need for psychotropic medications.

Specific inpatient units for persuasion are not necessary. Implementing persuasion-focused groups on short-term general inpatient psychiatry units is not complicated;[12] such a resource is important in managing dual diagnosis patients. Such groups have the additional benefit of helping psychiatric staff overcome their own feelings of powerlessness and discouragement about complex substance abusing patients. The group can form a focus of hope, allowing staff to know that they have truly done all that can be done.

Further study of the relative value of inpatient vs. outpatient, and individual vs. group, approaches to persuasion of dual diagnosis patients may be especially worthwhile. If persuasion is not effective treatment proceeds no further.

ACTIVE (PRIMARY) TREATMENT

This phase of treatment is intended to help patients develop the attitudes and skills needed to manage their chronic, potentially relapsing psychiatric and substance use disorders. In uncomplicated substance dependent patients, primary treatment has traditionally been offered in inpatient settings. There is ample evidence, however, that effective primary treatment for these patients can be delivered in the outpatient setting, and intensive outpatient treatment programs are becoming more common.

There are three reported open trials of outpatient peer group oriented treatments for dual diagnosis patients.[13,14,16] Kofoed et al.[13] reported on a highly structured sequential treatment approach, emphasizing abstinence and utilizing external structures and controls such as disulfiram (Antabuse) and urine drug screening. This approach had a drop-out rate no worse than that of primary substance dependence treated in the same facility. Patients who were engaged in treatment for three months or more had reduced hospital utilization compared to the year before specialized treatment. Substance use was markedly reduced in patients who completed treatment. Hellerstein and Meehan[14] reported on a less structured ongoing group for schizophrenic patients with a variety of substance use problems, including some on methadone maintenance. Their less structured approach also produced reductions in hospital utilization as well as reduced substance use, and had a lower dropout rate despite (or because of) a greater tolerance for alcohol/drug use during treatment. Hanson et al.,[16] reported a large open trial of a program for dual diagnosis patients with severe chronic mental illness. They provided conjoint treatment, comprehensive services, and encouraged involvement in self-help groups. They too reported improvements in substance use, psychiatric symptomatology, social functioning, and reduced rehospitalization. Like Kofoed et al.,[13] they used biochemical methods to detect relapse, and utilized brief psychiatric hospitalization if necessary.

Other authors have reported on inpatient programs which incorporate early treatment including primary treatment for dual diagnosis patients.[7,8] In theory at least, such programs offer the advantage of providing services including stabilization, engagement, persuasion, and primary treatment in a single efficient setting, avoiding the inevitable drop-out that comes with between-program transfers or the need to rely on general psychiatric units which may be inexpert and/or ambivalent about their role with dual diagnosis patients. Conversely, patients must be accepting of treatment before they will agree to be admitted onto such a unit. The presence of such units does not relieve general psychiatry wards of their responsibility to engage and persuade patients towards appropriate specialized treatment.

There are currently no studies, either controlled or uncontrolled, directly comparing the efficacy of inpatient vs. outpatient primary treatment for these dual diagnosis patients. While it seems reasonable that diagnosis or severity might promote a choice of inpatient vs. outpatient settings, available studies suggest that after stabilization extremely symptomatic patients with a variety of severe chronic psychiatric illnesses can be treated in outpatient programs. Thus differential treatment planning must be based on clinical judgment and social and ecological factors rather than data. While very disturbed and disadvantaged patients can receive effective primary treatment in an outpatient setting, such treatment requires access to a competent and cooperative inpatient psychiatry unit willing to deal with unremitting relapses of either condition.

I tend to favor a sequential treatment process, with escalating limits and rewards, and use of urine drug screening and pharmacologic aids to abstinence such as disulfiram or naltrexone. Despite my bias less structured approaches also appear helpful, do seem to produce benefit, and may retain patients in treatment who would be discharged from more structured programs. Though inpatient programs may be able to deliver needed skills more quickly and efficiently, major psychiatric illnesses such as schizophrenia limit the intensity of such programs, especially as compared to residential treatment for primary substance dependence.[1,3,7]

Further studies must define patient sub-populations who benefit differentially from these different approaches. These studies must utilize clearly described, standardized treatments. Examination of techniques to rate motivation for abstinence may also be productive. In primary substance dependence evidence suggests that professional staff can predict treatment completion with some success, but that patients are better able to predict the chances of post-treatment sobriety.[17] Ries et al.[8] have shown that dual diagnosis patient self-ratings of motivation for abstinence are significantly predictive of abstinence a month post hospital discharge. Such ratings may prove useful in assigning patients to the appropriate treatment stage (i.e., persuasion vs. primary treatment). They should not be used to arbitrarily exclude patients from treatment. Another potentially productive study area involves patient choice; at least one study in primary substance dependence suggests that offering patients treatment choices may improve treatment retention.[18] This should be specifically examined in dual diagnosis patients.

Throughout treatment plans must be *progressive* and *specific*. It is difficult to remain clear about the appropriate treatment stage assignment for a given patient, and challenging to implement specific sequential treatment offerings with a progressive incentive structure as patients proceed through treatment. A simple, useful way to assure that treatment interventions are specific and progressive is to periodically ask treatment staff this question: "If this patient takes the treatment step we have asked (for instance attending sessions regularly, or attaining several weeks of sobriety) what will be different in the treatment we will *then* offer him/her?" The answer to this question often makes clear either the strength or hollowness of incentives towards improvement; conversely difficulty in providing a clear answer demonstrates failure of the treatment plan to communicate direction and provide meaningful incentives to the patient.

RELAPSE PREVENTION (AFTERCARE)

Aftercare for primary substance dependent patients comprises supportive care to maintain the gains of primary treatment, including sobriety. Aftercare inevitably involves managing relapses to reduce their duration and destructiveness. In treatment of dual diagnosis patients, this approach to *managing* chronic disease extends to both the substance dependence and psychiatric illnesses.[3,7] The distinction between primary treatment and aftercare is blurred in dual diagnosis patients. Significant relapse of psychiatric illness may undo to an extent the benefits of primary treatment requiring repetition of primary treatment components, while slower integration of knowledge and skills during primary treatment requires a blurring of the primary treatment/aftercare boundary with extension of primary treatment into outpatient aftercare treatment.[3,7,13]

Relapse prevention concepts are applicable to both co-morbid illnesses. Relapse prevention involves identifying risk factors for relapse, warning signs of imminent relapse, and developing specific plans to minimize the damage of relapse (as opposed to catastrophizing relapse). Relapse must be treated as something to be avoided if possible, but given the basic chronic relapsing nature of these disorders it is clearly wisest to acknowledge the possibility of relapse and make it clear that relapse (within certain predetermined limits) will not lead to rejection or punishment.[3] There are some data[6,19] suggesting that relapse of either condition produces decompensation of other co-morbid disorders. Brief inpatient treatment on a general psychiatry ward minimizes the reverberating effects of relapse. It is essential that staff view such treatment as a legitimate part of their role, so that they will not be judgmental or rejecting.

Aftercare occurs predominantly in an outpatient setting; the days of leisurely and prolonged inpatient treatment are clearly passed, particularly in the absence of evidence of particular effectiveness. Relapse prevention techniques can be applied in individual treatment. Group treatment can be more efficient and is believed by many clinicians to be more effective, though controlled comparisons have not been done. Inpatient resources may be needed to minimize the effects of either psychiatric or substance dependence relapse.

Specialized aftercare units are probably not required. The controlled environment of a well-run general psychiatric unit, combined with prompt symptom control using appropriate psychotropic agents, is an effective support to ongoing outpatient aftercare.

PHARMACOLOGIC ADJUNCTS
TO OUTPATIENT TREATMENT SETTINGS

In both outpatient primary treatment and aftercare clinicians may utilize a variety of pharmacologic adjuncts focused specifically on substance abuse. Probably the best known and studied are disulfiram (Antabuse) which produces an aversive and occasionally dangerous reaction to alcohol ingestion; methadone and other long-acting opiate agonists, which have demonstrated efficacy in reducing illicit opiate use; and naltrexone (Trexan), a long-acting opiate antagonist which effectively blocks intoxication from opiate use. These adjuncts should not be considered sufficient treatment in themselves, but may be useful in supporting primary treatment on an outpatient basis, and in reducing the risk of relapse during aftercare.

Disulfiram has been extensively studied in primary alcoholics; remarkably enough it seems to contribute only modestly to treatment success. Despite the limited data supporting the value of disulfiram, many clinicians (including this author) have encountered individual patients who attribute their sobriety to use of disulfiram, and hence continue to see it as a useful adjunct. Clinicians are often advised to avoid disulfiram in dual diagnosis patients. Disulfiram does have the potential to exacerbate psychosis.[20] However most reports of symptom exacerbation are in unmedicated chronic patients given high disulfiram doses. Kofoed et al.[13] used disulfiram routinely in a small group of patients with psychotic illnesses *after* they were stabilized and maintained on appropriate psychotropic medications. They found that compliance with disulfiram therapy was as good in dual diagnosis[13] as in primary alcoholic outpatients.[21] They reported no particular difficulties, and concluded disulfiram seemed less of a risk than continued alcohol use. Controlled studies of the safety and efficacy of disulfiram in these patients are greatly needed.

Methadone itself seems to have some antipsychotic properties.[22] In patients who otherwise meet the criteria for eligibility for methadone maintenance treatment, psychosis is not a contraindication to concurrent use of methadone and diagnosis appropriate psychotropics. Methadone may enhance the possibilities for outpatient treatment of certain dually diagnosed patients with opiate dependence disorders.

Naltrexone is an interesting and potentially valuable agent. An opiate antagonist, it has been used in primary opiate dependence as a treatment adjunct with some benefit. It has also been examined as a treatment in several other psychiatric conditions. Specific study of this drug in dual diagnosis patients will be of great interest; however at this time its role is not clearly defined.

A variety of treatments have been examined to help manage cocaine dependence. Recent studies have examined various tricyclic antidepressants, amantadine, bromocriptine, carbamazepine, clonidine, and lithium as agents to diminish craving and relapse to cocaine use. Specific study of these agents in dual diagnosis patients has not been done. Given potential interactions between these treatments, psychotic illness, and antipsychotic medications, specific study of their safety and efficacy in dual diagnosis patients is needed.

CONCLUSION

Available data suggest that dual diagnosis patients can be treated with success rates similar to treatment of primary substance abusers. I suggest developing treatment plans in the context of sequential treatment stages, and have reviewed clinical factors which may effect treatment decisions at each stage.

We know little about which patient subpopulations may respond to different treatment approaches or settings. There are adequate data and suggestions about treatment planning to allow us to make necessary decisions in our ongoing clinical work, though there remains a lot of uncertainty about these decisions. Available experience and data leave much room for ongoing clinical innovation and evaluation.

REFERENCES

1. McLellan AT. Psychiatric severity as a predictor of outcome from substance abuse treatments. In: Meyer RE, ed. Psychopathology and Addictive Disorders. New York: Guilford Press, 1986:97-139.

2. Kofoed L. Assessment of comorbid psychiatric illness and substance disorders. In: Minkoff K, Drake RE eds. Dual Diagnosis of Major Mental Illness and Substance Disorder. New Directions for Mental Health Services number 50. San Francisco: Jossey-Bass Inc., 1991:43-55.

3. Osher FC, Kofoed LL. Treatment of patients with psychiatric and psychoactive substance abuse disorders. Hosp Comm Psychiatry 1989; 40:1025-30.

4. Pinsker H. Addicted patients in hospital psychiatric units. Psychiatric Annals 1983; 13:619-23.

5. Shore JH, Kofoed L. Community intervention in the treatment of alcoholism. Alcoholism Clin Exp Res 1984; 8:151-159.

6. Drake RE, Osher FC, Wallach MA. Alcohol use and abuse in schizophrenia: A prospective community study. J Nerv Ment Dis 1989; 177:408-14.

7. Minkoff K. An integrated treatment model for dual diagnosis of psychosis and addiction. Hosp Comm Psychiatry 1989; 40:1031-6.

8. Reis RK, Ellingson T. A pilot assessment at one month of seventeen dual diagnosis patients. Hosp Comm Psychiatry 1990; 41:1230-33.

9. Gelberg L, Linn LS, Leake BD. Mental health, alcohol and drug use, and criminal history among homeless adults. Am J Psychiatry 1988; 145:191-6.

10. Dolan LP. An intake group in the alcoholism outpatient clinic. J Stud Alcohol 1975; 36:996-9.

11. Stark MJ, Kane BJ. General and specific psychotherapy role induction with substance-abusing clients. Int J Addict 1985; 20:1135-41.

12. Kofoed L, Keys A. Using group therapy to persuade dual-diagnosis patients to seek substance abuse treatment. Hosp Comm Psychiatry 1988; 39: 1209-11.

13. Kofoed L, Kania J, Walsh T, et al. Outpatient treatment of patients with substance abuse and coexisting psychiatric disorders. Am J Psychiatry 1986; 143:867-872.

14. Hellerstein DJ, Meehan B. Outpatient group therapy for schizophrenic substance abusers. Am J Psychiatry 1987; 144:1337-9.

15. Atkinson RM. Persuading alcoholic patients to seek treatment. Comp Therapy 1985; 11:16-24.

16. Hanson M, Kramer TH, Gross W. Outpatient treatment of adults with coexisting substance use and mental disorders. J Substance Abuse Treatment 1990; 7:109-16.

17. Vanicelli M, Becker B. Prediction of outcome in treatment of alcoholism: A study of staff and patients. J Stud Alcohol 1981; 42:928-50.

18. Raymond JS, Hurwitz S. Client preference-treatment congrunce as a facilitator of length of stay: Supporting an old truism. Int J Addict 1981; 16:431-41.

19. Castaneda R, Galanter M, Lifshutz H, et al. Effect of drugs of abuse on psychiatric symptoms among hospitalized schizophrenics. Am J Drug Alcohol Abuse 1991; 17:313-320.

20. Major LF, Lerner P, Ballenger JC, et al. Dopamine beta-hydroxylase in the cerebrospinal fluid: Relationship to disulfiram-induced psychosis. Biol Psychiatry 1979; 14:337-44.

21. Kofoed LL. Chemical monitoring of disulfiram compliance: A study of alcoholic outpatients. Alcoholism Clin Exp Res 1987; 11:481-5.

22. Brizer DA, Hartman N, Sweeney J, et al. Effect of methadone plus neuroleptics on treatment-resistant chronic paranoid schizophrenia. Am J Psychiatry 1985; 142:1106-7.

An Integrated Psychology
for the Addictions:
Beyond the Self-Medication Hypothesis

R. Jeffrey Goldsmith, MD

SUMMARY. The Self-Medication Hypothesis (SMH) is a popular explanation for chemical dependencies. The SMH ignores or leaves out important biological research which has explored the mechanisms of reward, motivation to use alcohol/drugs, as well as the impact on mood of chronic, excessive alcohol/drug use. A new psychology is needed which includes this biological research as well as the psychological observations contained in the SMH. Self Psychology is used to create an integrated psychology for the addictions.

INTRODUCTION

Despite a compelling amount of relevant research over the last thirty to forty years supporting the disease concept of alcoholism

---

R. Jeffrey Goldsmith is affiliated with the Department of Psychiatry, College of Medicine, University of Cincinnati, 3259 Elland Avenue, Cincinnati, OH 45267-0539.

Requests for reprints should be addressed to Dr. Goldsmith.

[Haworth co-indexing entry note]: "An Integrated Psychology for the Addictions: Beyond the Self-Medication Hypothesis." Goldsmith, R. Jeffrey. Co-published simultaneously in *Journal of Addictive Diseases,* (The Haworth Press, Inc.) Vol. 12, No. 3, 1993, pp. 139-154; and: *Comorbidity of Addictive and Psychiatric Disorders* (Ed: Norman S. Miller, and Barry Stimmel) The Haworth Press, Inc., 1993, pp. 139-154. Multiple copies of this article/chapter may be purchased from The Haworth Document Delivery Center. Call 1-800-3-HAWORTH (1-800-342-9678) between 9:00 - 5:00(EST) and ask for DOCUMENT DELIVERY CENTER.

139

and elegantly exploring the biology of alcohol/drug addiction, the Self Medication Hypothesis (SMH) for addictive disorders still flourishes in the minds of many therapists.[1,2] This theory postulates that the motivation to consume alcohol or other drugs of addiction in substantial quantities over a long period of time is to "medicate" a dysthymic, anxious, or psychotic state. There are several parts to this hypothesis which need to be assessed in order to ascertain its validity. The first is the motivation to drink or use drugs for a chemically dependent individual. Second is the implications of the word "medicate," and the third is the rationale that the purpose of the use is to change an unpleasant mood, to alleviate stress, or to respond to some uncomfortable tension. This paper will review the major points of the SMH, what it overlooks, and why it is not helpful in the treatment of addictive disorders. A self psychological understanding will be integrated with the biological research observations to develop a more comprehensive biopsychosocial understanding of alcoholism and drug addiction relevant to diagnosis and treatment.

WHAT THE SELF-MEDICATION HYPOTHESIS OVERLOOKS

The SMH emphasizes the psychological motivation for alcohol/drug use.[3] The need to reduce emotional suffering is considered the primary motivation to use, while pleasure-seeking or stimulus-seeking motives are considered by-products, secondary to the problems of self-regulation.[4] Implicit in the name SMH is the concept of prescribing medication. Khantzian says "individuals prefer or depend on different drugs because each class of drugs, much like the classes of drugs legitimately used in psychiatry, have a distinctive action and effect which interacts with specific painful feeling states and related psychiatric disorders."[5] Distress and suffering are at the heart of alcoholism and addiction, and the SMH takes into consideration how the class of drugs chosen interacts with the distress. Other factors, including genetic, environmental, and cultural variables, are considered modifiers of the individual's vulnerability to alcohol/drug addiction. Loss of control is not a central problem, it is psychological regression brought about by the long-term use of alcohol/drugs.[6] The SMH emphasizes the "enduring and relatively immutable personality structures" which have created long-standing difficulties intraphysically and interpersonally.

There are several important issues to highlight in the SMH. First, the most important motivation is the person's need to relieve distress. Second, this is done in a specific fashion, by choosing a particular drug for its particular drug effect, much the way a physician chooses his prescription. Third, life turmoil is more the result of the psychological deficits than alcohol/drug induced behaviors, and the biological effects of alcohol/drug use are secondary factors.

What is at stake is important–the patient's life and the family. The SMH would dictate that therapy be focused on the psychological deficits which are considered the heart of the matter. It suggests that there is a purpose to the alcohol/drug use–to quiet the internal distress much the way a doctor would. If chronic, excessive alcohol/drug use renders the individual more depressed, anxious, or psychotic, then the SMH would conclude that continued use stemmed from a too severe problem that needs greater medication. Furthermore, likening chronic alcohol/drug use to a physician's prescription discourages the therapist from calling a halt to the alcohol/drug dependency because it is viewed as therapeutic, as relieving suffering.

The first point, relief of distress, fails to distinguish whether this is a dysphoric mood and symptom or a biological syndrome. The former is an affective state, such as sadness, which everyone experiences from time to time. Alcohol and CNS depressant drugs can induce feelings of sadness. This has been demonstrated experimentally with nonalcoholic volunteers,[7] as well as alcoholic subjects.[8,9] The intensity of this phenomenon depends upon the mood of the drinker as well as the amount of alcohol consumed and the context of the drinking episode.[10] In fact, the vast amount (98%) of alcoholics admitted to a residential unit expressed the mood of sadness; while 69% of those admitted to a hospital unit had moderate to severe depression as measured by a Hamilton or Zung Depression scale.[11] However, only 8.6% of them met clinical criteria for depressive disorder. This is of critical importance because the treatment of major depressive disorder is quite different from the treatment of an alcohol/drug induced mood disorder. The latter is effectively treated by maintaining abstinence from the drug, while the depressive illness is treated most effectively with medications, ECT, or psychotherapy.

The amount of alcohol or drugs consumed as well as chronicity of consumption is another important factor which is often left out of the SMH. The research by Tamerin and Mendelson reported that alcoholics under experimental conditions did feel some relief and momentary improvement in their mood along with their first few drinks; however, as their drinking continued, the mood changed, often quite dramatically, to a morose or even suicidal state.[12] Contrary to the popular myth that alcoholics/addicts are having fun, they aren't. What starts out one way, ends up another. This has considerable clinical importance. It is insufficient clinically to focus on the first few drinks because this ignores the loss of control, the hangover, as well as the intrapsychic and interpersonal turmoil in response to the morbid drunkenness. This is acknowledged by Khantzian, Wurmser, and others but not integrated into their psychology of addiction. The need for abstinence to reverse the alcohol/drug induced complications must have a central part in a treatment paradigm.

Loss of control is widely recognized and typical for many alcoholics and drug addicts.[13] The alcoholic/addict has an illusion that he can control alcohol/drugs. Studies with animals have shown that certain drugs like cocaine and morphine, when injected into the nucleus accumbens and ventral tegmentum respectively, lead to compulsive self-administration.[14] The literature suggests that there is a "reward" area in the brain which triggers this repetitive self-administration. Animals develop a behavior of persistent self-administration with cocaine and opiates much the way crack users and intravenous drug users behave.[15] The SMH suggests that such persistent behavior will go away with the right interpretation and support. The research suggests that there is a biologically driven compulsion which over-rides normal habits.

The chronicity of drug or alcohol use is important for several reasons. Clinical studies suggest that cocaine depletes the brain of catecholamines after repetitive use and that dopamine depletion specifically seems to be associated with an intense desire for more drug.[16] Since, in animals, the rewarding effects of amphetamine and cocaine appear to be mediated through the mesolimbic dopamine system,[17] it is likely that this area is responsible for the strong reinforcing properties and that depletion of dopamine in the nucleus accumbens leads to this urge to use.[18] Both drug reinforcement and the post-use urges are powerful biological motivators.[19]

In addition to the depletion theory of chronic cocaine use, other researchers[20] have shown that conditioned responses may produce a strong urge to use the drug. Childress et al. have shown that desensitization treatment of these conditioned responses for the addicts who exhibit strong physiological symptoms of withdrawal along with a desire to use the drug in response to environmental cues (which trigger the addict to think about using drugs) will improve the relapse rates.[21] Such conditioned responses are thought to play a role in situational urges for drug use for over 40% of the addicts. This urge to use can lead to major setbacks and relapse to compulsive drug use.[22] The biological and physiological theories of these conditioned responses are essential to a thorough understanding of the motivation to use psychoactive drugs. The last decade has produced considerable research on the nature of these triggers and therapists have developed techniques to intervene effectively with them.[23]

Combining what we know about the nucleus accumbens and ventral tegmental areas with the biology of these conditioned responses, gives us a very important motivational system which appears to be biologically driven and perhaps drug induced.[24] With lab animals, only very palatable foods and sex-related stimuli seem capable of activating the mesolimbic system with the near potency of the drug-induced motivation from the ventral tegmental area or nucleus accumbens. It's important to note that morphine, nicotine, and Cannabis also activate this system with somewhat less potency reflecting the addictive potential of these drugs in human usage. A model for chemical dependency must include these potent biological drives as well as the initial motivation to use the drugs which are probably psychosocial in nature.

The idea of "self-medicating" a dysphoric mood state has been tested through the research literature. There have been several major experiments in the last thirty years which clarified the nature of drug and alcohol use by people with dysphoric moods. The concept of self-medicating a dysphoric mood incorporates the idea that somebody is distressed and uses the drug to feel better. As mentioned previously, experimental subjects actually felt worse when consuming large quantities of alcohol, regardless of how they felt at the beginning of the experiment.[25] Mayfield and Coleman showed that there are a variety of changes in drinking in response to an affective swing among bipolar and unipolar patients.[26] They looked at affective disordered patients with histories of excessive drinking and found that more than half of the patients did not change their drinking patterns in response to mood change. Moreover, they found that all (N = 19) manic patients increased their drinking, whereas depressed patients tended to decrease their drinking more often (10 of 16) than increase it. Studies that look at the impact of antidepressants in the treatment of alcoholism have shown unpromising results. All the studies with a controlled design demonstrated no beneficial effects when antidepressants were used with alcoholics.[27] Studies that look at the rate of alcoholism among patients with major depressive disorder have shown that only five to ten percent of patients with primary major depressive disorders actually develop alcoholism, and a causal link between depression and subsequent alcoholism is not established.[28]

Findings are quite similar when major anxiety disorders are studied. Four major studies with anxious patients meeting criteria for phobia, panic disorder, and agoraphobia have shown that ten to twenty percent meet the diagnostic criteria for alcoholism.[29-32] These are all consistent with or somewhat lower than the national average for alcoholism.[33]

Studies have looked at the choices which humans make when offered a choice of drugs. These drugs which are known to have an addictive liability (e.g., opiates, stimulants, nicotine, anxiolytics/sedatives, alcohol, and marijuana) have all been self-administered by humans in laboratories.[34] In contrast, a variety of drugs which have little or no known addiction liability (e.g., neuroleptics, nonstimulants anorectics, and antihistamines) do not act as reinforcers. Under standardized laboratory conditions drugs like alcohol and amphetamine cause some healthy volunteers a dysphoric feeling which leads to avoidance.[35] When anxious volunteers (N = 24) and healthy volunteers (N = 12) were offered diazepam in 5mg doses, 21 of 36 subjects did not choose the active drug or did so only once.

When they were offered placebo or 10mg doses, 27 of 36 did not choose active drug or did so only once, despite reporting less anxiety. In contrast, when amphetamine was offered these subjects, 10 of 36 subjects chose it 2-3 times and 20 of 36 chose it 4-5 times. There was no difference between the anxious groups and the control group with regard to their choice for either diazepam or amphetamines. Other studies by deWit et al. have shown that subjects with histories of drug addiction were likely to choose benzodiazepines whereas controls were not.[36] These findings suggest that, with anxiolytics, it is a history of drug addiction that predicts choice, not anxiety. This reflects the low addiction liability for benzodiazepines. Amphetamines, on the other hand, are chosen by many anxious and healthy volunteers. This suggests that it is the drug effect which is desirable, not the relief from an uncomfortable state.

If we look at the issue of dysphoric mood as a characterological problem, we come up with similar results. There appears to be a myth that alcoholism is generated because of an unhappy and unstable childhood. A prospective study done by Vaillant et al. suggested that there were not any differences between the alcoholic and nonalcoholic adults when their childhood was examined for emotional disturbance, family problems, or school performance.[37] There didn't seem to be any differences in the mother-child relationships. As a matter of fact, the authors began to wonder if the alcoholics might not exaggerate their childhood difficulties in order to explain their adult problems. A different prospective study undertaken by McCord and McCord found that dependent and oral tendencies of the boys did not predict future alcoholism.[38] They found that, contrary to popular belief, the boys who later became alcoholic men were outwardly confident, less disturbed by fears, more aggressive and active, and more heterosexual. Such findings do not seem to support the SMH.

A new field in psychology is the study of the drinkers' expectancies about alcohol as a way of predicting drinking behaviors. Questionnaires measuring the drinkers' expectancies regarding certain aspects of alcohol's effects on behavior, mood and emotions have been developed.[39] The scales look at expectancies about sexual behaviors, assertiveness, pleasure, tension reduction, aggression, nasty effects, impairment in functioning, disinhibition, gregariousness, and depressant effects. The scales do predict drinking behaviors to some extent; however, the scales only explain 10-20% of the variance regarding frequency of episodes, quantity consumed, frequency of intoxication, and overall drinking. More importantly the sex and age of the drinker, as well as the attitudes about drinking and getting drunk explain a greater amount of the variance than expectancies explain.

There are probably multiple reasons why such professional myths and stereotypes continue to be maintained. Unfortunately, the legacy of what we learned from our teachers whom we esteem and value is very difficult to alter. Many studies have shown that professionals do not enjoy working with alcoholics/addicts which suggests that clinicians might not continue to study or learn about such a patient population.[40] It has been well documented that the substance use disorders have not been amply or well taught in professional training.[41] In addition, there is considerable confusion clinically between the primary mood disorders (e.g., manic depressive illness, major depressive disorder, and the anxiety disorders) and the organic mental disorders. The phenomenology is virtually identical and the only way to differentiate them is to take a careful history, have a high titer of suspicion, do drug testing, and be willing to wait a period of time when the patient is abstinent, to see if the symptoms go away without any pharmacological intervention. Moreover, the sedative/alcohol withdrawal states exhibit symptoms that are quite similar to some of the symptoms of anxiety disorders. Without taking a careful history and getting corroboration from an outside source, a clinician could easily mistake a mild sedative withdrawal for a primary anxiety disorder.

The typical defenses displayed by alcoholics and drug addicts frequently obscure the real drug and alcohol history of the person at hand.[42] The mixture of denial, disavowal, rationalization, projection, etc. makes it quite difficult for a counselor or a psychotherapist to differentiate the causal connection of thought, feeling, and action from the compulsively driven behavior of the addictive cycle. The validity of alcohol and drug histories has historically been shown to be very low. Studies with alcoholics[43] and drug addicts[44] have shown that about 50% of alcoholics' histories and 80% of drug histories can be disproved by a timely drug screen.

PSYCHOLOGY OF AN INTEGRATED MODEL

There is growing evidence and a growing consensus that alcoholism is a complex biopsychosocial syndrome.[45] Such a model is based upon the genetics of alcoholism and drug addiction which includes the inheritance of factors such as tolerance and the propensity for withdrawal symptoms.[46,47] Researchers have described the biology of reinforcement, neurotransmitter depletion, and even a protracted abstinence syndrome.[48] Failure to include these biological findings removes the power, elegance and relevance behind a psychology which could help us understand the drug addict and alcoholic more completely. Furthermore, a psychology which ignores the biology of addictive disorders loses its capacity to describe such complex syndromes. The psychology which integrates the biological findings with the experience of the individual will not only help the clinician understand the plight of the addict, but it will also prove to be more effective clinically. The interventions will be more accurate and will be received with more recognition and acceptance by the patient.

Such a psychology needs to incorporate the individual's experience of the biological phenomena of addiction, such as tolerance, loss of control, craving, denial, withdrawal symptoms, and the changes in personality sequelae of alcohol/drug addiction which include the organic mood disorders, organic anxiety disorders, as well as the protracted abstinence syndrome (sleep disturbances, labile affect, and anhedonia). Such a psychology is not an intuitively logical model, but a model which helps us understand the experience of the chemically dependent individual. Such a model must help us conceptualize denial and show us how to make a proper intervention. Such a model must be able to incorporate the family members and extended social networks which are typically included in the descriptions of the family system of the chemically dependent family. It would be imperative for this psychology to help us understand the phenomenon of co-dependency which has become such an important concept in psychotherapy and rehabilitation counseling in recent years.[49]

The new psychoanalytic theory of self psychology is experience-near and relies heavily upon the empathic vantage point for collect-

ing data as well as the empathic connection for its healing trans-
formations.[50,51] The self is considered the primary psychological
experience of the individual while the attainment of psychological
wholeness and the maintenance of that cohesion are the primary
psychological motivations.[52] The self can maintain this important
homeostasis for healthy narcissism through a complex network of
important relationships which are called self self-object (SSO) relationships. Implied in this concept is the experience that these other
people are part of oneself, are providing critical self-regulatory
functions which the individual cannot yet do for himself independently.[53] Repeated breaks with or frustrations by the self-object
disrupt the SSO relationship and lead to a hunger for a reliable and
predictable self-object. Continued SSO disruptions are painful experiences leaving the person feeling shattered or unglued. People who
experience such fragmentation are often overwhelmed, suicidal, or
enraged. If such a person seeks reassurance from alcohol/drugs, he
is vulnerable to develop such a SSO relationship. Alcohol and
drugs, initially, appear easy to control and very reliable. This is not
a causative motivation but a highly reinforcing motivation. Such
vulnerability is typical with narcissistic pathology[54] and accounts
for the self-deficits described by the SMH.[55]

Critical for an integrated psychology is the self experience of the
loss of control over alcohol/drug use, described by Alcoholics
Anonymous.[56] For drugs like crack this unmanageability and loss
of control could come suddenly; and for others, like alcohol, it
occurs over a long period of time. The self would experience these
two situations somewhat differently and would respond accordingly. The intense pleasure of crack and the depression and desire for
cocaine in withdrawal continues to drive the person to use, despite
the fears and anxieties about losing control. While the dynamics
resemble SMH, it is important to appreciate that this is drug-induced.
This occurs early in the process of cocaine addiction which would
produce a highly ambivalent crack user who felt out of control but
still wanted to use the drug very much. Treatment dropouts and
frequent relapses would be expected. On the other hand, the alcoholic frequently drinks for years before he gets into treatment. The
process of losing control and reestablishing some stability, only to
relapse and lose control again, leads to a slightly different self

experience. The alcoholic has more time to make excuses and set up an elaborate system of disavowal which becomes a major barrier to recovery.[57] Furthermore, the alcoholic often goes through periods where he tries to control his life without giving up drinking alcohol altogether.[58] Only when these attempts at controlling things have been exhausted can the alcoholic surrender to the inevitable idea that he has control over drinking no longer. AA describes this process as "being sick and tired of being sick and tired." It's not surprising that such an individual would be exhausted, depleted, and bewildered when he reached a therapist.

There is an additional self experience which is crucial to the understanding of the chemically dependent individual and important to incorporate into the treatment process. The experience of losing control is a frightening and traumatic experience for the self. The realization and acceptance of this is frequently so painful that defenses ward off the full impact. It is the acceptance of such a scary reality which becomes the focus of AA, as well as recovery-oriented treatment programs.[59] The self psychological understanding of addictions would focus on this too. The psychological defense of disavowal allows the alcoholic or drug addict the capacity to deny the implications of his own behaviors which he does perceive to a certain extent. With disavowal, however, the material is not unconscious, behind the repression barrier. It is more accessible to consciousness, and hence therapy. The use of empathy in understanding the person and as a tool for interpretive interventions facilitates this process of reconnecting the disavowed material.[60]

The person who is dependent does not understand and did not intend the biological idiosyncrasies and changes that occur with drinking/drug taking. The chemically dependent individual thinks that he is in charge of his life and that he is making decisions. The chemically dependent person's good intentions, to control drinking/drug use as well as have a good time, appear to go awry as the illness progresses and the behavior becomes more out of control and unmanageable as a result of the heavy drug use/drinking binges. The person is frustrated and enraged at his inability to make things happen the way he intends.[61,62] Until the biological loss of control is understood, the person cannot put into proper perspective what is happening; and, consequently, he blames himself. It is only when the alcoholic/addict accepts that things are out of control that he can understand how to regain a healthy balance in mood and relationships through a commitment to abstinence. For those who arrive at such acceptance after a long struggle with numerous defeats and personal loses, there is a traumatic loss of confidence in the self's capacity to direct and guide the individual through life. It is not uncommon for recovering individuals to seek reassurance and guidance from mentors, support groups like Alcoholics Anonymous, or therapists. By developing SSO relationships with such people and institutions, the person can settle himself down and develop some confidence that he knows how to organize himself in a safe and productive manner. The development of such confidence and competence takes a number of years and should not be considered a quick and easily obtained product of therapy. A recovery-oriented psychotherapy as described by Brown[63] and others[64] will provide the necessary abstinence for biological recovery by focusing on the need to stay completely sober. A self psychological understanding of the individual and his situation will facilitate the psychological recovery from the traumatic experience of having one's life deteriorate so dramatically. For those who came from dysfunctional families, the treatment of these self-deficits will be essential.

The self psychological understanding of the SSO relationship can also be used to understand and facilitate recovery from co-dependency. Because the immature self is reliant upon SSO relationships for a feeling of wholeness, the individual is vulnerable to the feedback from the significant others. Frustration by the self-object will lead to distress and self blame, often followed by trying to get the self-object to respond again. If the person who is used as a self-object is addicted to alcohol/drugs, he is bound to be frustrating and respond inappropriately. This interpersonal dynamic is central in the understanding of co-dependency, and this can be included in treatment whenever warranted.

Several themes have been identified by therapists who specialize in the psychotherapy of substance abusers.[65] Many people have identified the deficits or difficulties in mood-regulation, self-esteem maintenance, and self-care lifestyle behaviors. Deficits in these sectors can become developmental arrests in childhood, consistent with the experience of many chemically dependent adult children of alcoholics. However, a lifetime of alcohol/drug addiction can also inhibit development and cause developmental lags based upon deficits in adult development. Either way the centrality of the SSO relationship makes it an important concept in the long term recovery from these devastating illnesses. A focus on sobriety and abstinence, grounded in the understanding of the biological reward mechanisms, will provide the foundations for a new lifestyle. Such a psychology not only includes the biological research ignored by the SMH, but also the same psychological observations incorporated by the SMH. It gives insight into the distress experienced by the alcoholic/addict during treatment and facilitates a strong treatment alliance through an empathic connection. The dynamic understanding of self psychology suggests how to manage the development of SSO relationships, whether alcoholic/addict or family members. Such a new psychology should give us a more comprehensive theory of addictive disorders plus have the capacity to incorporate new biological research.

REFERENCES

1. Khantzian EJ. Self-regulation and self-medication factors in alcoholism and the addictions: similarities and differences. In: Galanter M. ed. Recent developments in alcoholism. Vol. 8. New York: Plenum Press. 1990: 255-271.

2. Rado S. The psychoanalysis of pharmacothymia (drug addiction).J Sub Abuse Treatment. 1984; 1: 59-68.

3. Khantzian EJ. *op.cit.*

4. Khantzian EJ. *op.cit.*, p.256.

5. Khantzian EJ. *op.cit.*, p.256.

6. Khantzian EJ. *op.cit.*, p.259.

7. Warren GH, & Raynes AE. Mood changes during three conditions of alcohol intake. Quart J Stud Alc. 1972; 3: 979-989.

8. Mayfield DG, and Coleman LL. Alcohol use and affective disorder. Disease of the Nervous System. 1968, July: 467-474.

9. Tamerin JS, and Mendelson JH. The psychodynamics of chronic inebriation: observations of alcoholics during the process of drinking in an experimental group setting. Am J Psychiatry. 1969; 125: 886-899.

10. Schuckit MA. Alcoholism and affective disorder: diagnostic confusion. In: Goodwin DW, Erickson CK. eds. Alcoholism and affective disorders. New York: SP Medical Scientific Books, 1979: 9-19.

11. Keeler MH, Taylor CI, and Miller WC. Are all recently detoxified alcoholics depressed? Am J Psychiatry. 1979; 136: 586-588.

12. Tamerin JS, Mendelson JH. *op.cit.*

13. Vaillant GE. The course of alcoholism and lessons for treatment. In: Grinspoon L. ed. Psychiatry update. Vol. III. Washington, DC: American Psychiatric Press, Inc. 1984: 311-319.

14. Wise RA. The brain and reward. In: Liebman JM, Cooper SJ. eds. The neuropharmacology of reward. Oxford: Oxford University Press, 1989.

15. Wise RA. *op.cit.*

16. Washton AM. Cocaine addiction. New York: W.W. Norton & Company, 1989.

17. Wise RA. *op.cit.*

18. Koob GF, and Bloom FE. Cellular and Molecular mechanisms of drug dependence. Science. 1988; 242: 715-723.

19. Wise RA. *op.cit.*

20. Litman GK. Stress, affect and craving in alcoholics. Quart J Stud Alc. 1974; 35:131-146.

21. Childress AR, McLellan AT, & O'Brien CP. Measurement and extinction of conditioned withdrawal-like responses in opiate-dependent patients. In: Problems of Drug Dependence 1983. Rockville: U.S. Department of Health and Human Services. 1984: 212-219.

22. Childress *et al. op.cit.*

23. Eds. Marlatt GA, and Gordon JR. Relapse Prevention. New York: The Guilford Press, 1985.

24. Wise RA. *op.cit.*

25. Tamerin JS, Mendelson JH. *op.cit.*

26. Mayfield DG, Coleman LL. *op.cit.*

27. Schuckit MA. *op.cit.*

28. Schuckit MC, and Monteiro MG. Alcoholism, anxiety and depression. Br J Addiction. 1988; 83: 1373-1380.

29. Marks IM, Bailey JR, & Gelder MG. Modified leucotomy in severe agoraphobia: a controlled serial inquiry. Br J Psychiatry. 1966; 112: 757-769.

30. Quitkin FM, Rifkin A, Kaplan J, Klein DF, & Oaks G. Phobic anxiety syndrome complicated by drug dependence and addiction. Arch Gen Psychiatry. 1972; 27: 159-162.

31. Bibb JL, & Chambliss DL. Alcohol use and abuse among diagnosed agoraphobics. Behavior Research and Therapy. 1986; 24: 49-58.

32. Cloninger CR, Martin RL, Clayton P, & Guze B. A blind follow-up and family study of anxiety neurosis: preliminary analysis of the St. Louis 500. In: Klein DF, Rabkin J. eds. Anxiety: new research and changing concepts. New York: Raven Press, 1981.

33. Robins LN, Helzer JE, Weissman MM, Orvaschel H, Gruenberg E, Burke JD Jr, Regier DA. Lifetime prevalence of specific psychiatric disorders in three sites. Arch Gen Psychiatry. 1984; 41: 949-958.

34. deWit H. Preference procedures for testing the abuse liability of drugs in humans. Br J Addictions. in press.

35. deWit H, Uhlenhuth EH, Hedeker D, McCracken SG, and Johnson CE. Lack of preference for diazepam in anxious volunteers. Arch Gen Psychiatry. 1986; 43: 533-541.

36. deWit H. *op.cit.*

37. Vaillant GE. *op.cit.*

38. McCord W, & McCord J. Origins of Alcoholism. Stanford: Stanford University Press, 1960.

39. Leigh BC. Attitudes and expectancies as predictors of drinking habits: a comparison of three scales. J Stud Alc. 1989; 50: 432-440.

40. Group for the Advancement of Psychiatry. Substance Abuse Disorder: a psychiatric priority. Am J Psychiatry. 148: 1291-300.

41. Health Professions Education. Alcohol Health & Research World. 1989; 13: 6-67.

42. Zweben JE. Recovery-oriented psychotherapy: patient resistances and therapist dilemmas. J Sub Ab Treatment. 1989; 6: 23-132.

43. Orrego H, Blake JE, Blendis LM, Kapur BM, and Isreal Y. Reliability of assessment of alcohol intake based on personal interviews in a liver clinic. Lancet. 1979; December: 1354-1356.

44. Ungerleider T, Lundberg GD, Sunshine I, and Walberg CB. The drug abuse warning network (DAWN) program. Arch Gen Psychiatry. 1989; 37: 106-109.

45. Meyer RE, and Babor TF. Explanatory models of alcoholism In: Tasman A, Hales RE, Frances AJ. eds. Review of psychiatry. vol. 8. Washington, DC.: American Psychiatric Press, Inc. 1989: 273-292.

46. Cloninger CR, Dinwiddie SH, and Reich T. Epidemiology and genetics of alcoholism. In: Tasman A, Hales RE, Frances AJ. eds. Review of psychiatry. vol. 8 Washington, D.C.: American Psychiatric Press, Inc. 1989: 293-308.

47. Bloom FE. Neurobiology of alcohol action and alcoholism. In: Tasman A, Hales RE, Frances AJ. eds. Review of psychiatry. Vol. 8. Washington, D.C.: American Psychiatric Press, Inc. 1989: 309-322.

48. Bloom FE. *op.cit.*

49. Cermak TL. Evaluating and treating adult children of alcoholics. Vol. 1 and vol. 2. Minneapolis: Johnson Institute, 1991.

50. Kohut H. How does analysis cure? Chicago: The University of Chicago Press, 1985.

51. Ornstein PH, and Kay J. Development of psychoanalytic self psychology: a historical-conceptual overview. In: Tasman A, Goldfinger SM, Kaufmann CA. Washing, D.C.: American Psychiatric Press, Inc., 1990: 303-322.

52. Kohut H. Thoughts on narcissism and narcissistic rage. In: Ornstein PH. ed. The search for the self-selected writings of Heing Kohut: 1950-1978. vol. 2. New York: International Universities. 1978: 615-658.

53. Orstein PH, Kay J. *op. cit.*

54. Kohut H. 1985. *op. cit.*

55. Khantzian EJ, Halliday KS, McAuliffe WE. Addiction and the vulnerable self. New York: Guilford Press, 1990.

56. Alcoholics anonymous. ed. 3rd. New York: Alcoholics Anonymous World Services, Inc., 1976.

57. Goldsmith RJ, Green BL. A rating scale for alcoholic denial. J Nerv Mental Disease. 1988; 176: 614-620.

58. Tiebout HM. The problem of gaining cooperation from the alcoholic patient. Quart J Stud Alc. 1947-48; 8: 47-54.

59. Brown S. Treating the alcoholic: a developmental model of recovery. New York: John Wiley & Sons, 1985.

60. Ornstein PH, Ornstein A. Clinical understanding and explaining: The empathic vantage point. In: Goldberg A. ed. Progress for self psychology. vol.1 New York: Guilford Press, 1985: 43-61.

61. Kohut H. 1978. *op. cit.*

62. Dodes LM. Addiction, helplessness, and narcissistic rage. Psychoanalytic Quar. 1990; LIX: 398-419.

63. Brown S. *op. cit.*

64. Zweben JE. Recovery oriented psychotherapy. J Sub Ab Treatment. 1986; 3: 255-262.

65. Khantzian EJ *et al. op. cit.*

Pharmacotherapy
of Psychiatric Syndromes
with Comorbid Chemical Dependence

David R. Gastfriend, MD

SUMMARY. Because of the paucity of research on the pharmacotherapy of psychiatric syndromes with comorbid psychoactive substance use disorders, treatment guidelines are primarily drawn from
general principles of clinical psychopharmacology and the addictive
disease model. Effective treatment requires the determination of a
discrete psychiatric diagnosis or working differential, consideration
of the range of drug effects as they vary over time, and awareness of
potential pharmacologic interactions between medication and alcohol or drug use. Either nonspecific prescribing or failure to treat may
result in protracted dysfunction, relapse, or medical morbidity and
mortality. Pharmacotherapy may also determine whether treatment

David R. Gastfriend is affiliated with the Department of Psychiatry, Harvard
Medical School, the Psychiatry Service of the Massachusetts General Hospital,
the Harvard-McLean Alcohol and Drug Abuse Research Center, and the Alcohol
and Chemical Dependence Rehabilitation Unit of the Spaulding Rehabilitation
Hospital.

Reprint requests should be addressed to Dr. David R. Gastfriend, Chief, Addiction Services, Massachusetts General Hospital, ACC-812, Fruit Street, Bos-
ton, MA 02114.

[Haworth co-indexing entry note]: "Pharmacotherapy of Psychiatric Syn-
dromes with Comorbid Chemical Dependence." Gastfriend, David R. Co-pub-
lished simultaneously in *Journal of Addictive Diseases,* (The Haworth Press,
Inc.) Vol. 12, No. 3, 1993, pp. 155-170; and: *Comorbidity of Addictive and
Psychiatric Disorders* (Ed: Norman S. Miller, and Barry Stimmel) The Haworth
Press, Inc., 1993, pp. 155-170. Multiple copies of this article/chapter may be
purchased from The Haworth Document Delivery Center. Call 1-800-3-
HAWORTH (1-800-342-9678) between 9:00 - 5:00(EST) and ask for DOC-
UMENT DELIVERY CENTER.

results in mere abstinence vs. recovery from addictive disease. Primary emphasis on non-pharmacologic strategies and the use of a formal treatment contract increase the likelihood of successful pharmacotherapy outcome.

INTERACTIONS BETWEEN ACUTE AND CHRONIC ALCOHOL/DRUG USE AND COMORBID PSYCHIATRIC SYNDROMES

Effective pharmacotherapy of the psychiatric syndrome in a dually diagnosed patient must consider several fundamental issues:[1] Does the patient actually have a discrete psychiatric diagnosis or is there at least a working differential, contingent upon further evidence and reevaluation?[2] What are the psychological and behavioral effects of the drug(s) being used by the patient?[3] What is the patient's temporal state of substance use, along the continuum of intoxication, withdrawal, cognitive impairment, abstinence and recovery.[4] Finally, what are the interactions between the chemical dependence and psychopharmacotherapy?[1]

Firm guidelines for pharmacotherapy of the dually diagnosed patient are limited by the paucity of available research. In this relative vacuum, chemical dependence workers criticize the trend toward "research dependence" overtaking common sense. It is worthwhile to recall how writers in medicine and psychiatry in the late 1970s colluded with the myth of cocaine's safety due to a lack of experimental data, rejecting enormous historical evidence to the contrary.

Clinical lore does exist in the literature, but disagreement abounds. In the extreme, opinions range from what Klerman has dubbed "pharmacologic Calvanism" (the view among many social model proponents being "the only good drug is a dead drug"), to "pharmacologic Hedonism" (or "better living through chemistry"). While interesting and useful for generating discussion, in actual practice these polar approaches pose many risks for patients. Proponents of the former view, such as therapeutic communities and social model programs, may influence patients to reject psychotropics altogether or decrease doses. Conversely, recovering persons often attest to experiences with iatrogenic substitute dependencies, such as a benzodiazepine for alcohol.

Some psychiatrists utilize a strategy in which reinforcing agents are prescribed to an actively dependent patient to achieve a "pill transference"–essentially an attempt to attach a handle to a hard-to-hold patient. Until a body of objective longitudinal studies emerges, the clinical experience of the practitioner and his/her trusted colleagues remains the standard of practice. Sample bias is a confounding factor, however, since the clinical expertise of each provider is constrained by the unique population to which he/she has been exposed. Thus, the psychiatrist working with a general chemical dependence population will experience different comorbidity prevalences, problems, and outcomes than one who primarily sees an affective and anxiety disorders practice.

Utility of Pharmacologic Principles

Pharmacologic properties of pharmacokinetics and pharmacodynamics become helpful in understanding the benefits and risks of drug therapies in the dual diagnosis population. The rate of onset of an agent's effect is a critical factor determining degree of reinforcement. Agents with routes of administration that produce rapid absorption, such as nicotine and cocaine, are therefore among the most addicting. Some patients have learned this for themselves, chewing alprazolam and lorazepam to achieve more rapid sublingual absorption and increasing their dependence, as a result. Another pharmacokinetic concern is the rate of transfer across the blood-brain barrier. Although all the benzodiazepines are relatively lipophilic, specific agents may vary by as much as 50-fold. For this reason, diazepam poses risks because of the "rush" it produces, in contrast to an agent such as chlordiazepoxide.

Pharmacodynamic properties may be important as well. Benzodiazepine dependence is not due to pharmacokinetic tolerance (i.e., there is no induction of metabolism) but rather pharmacodynamic tolerance (decreased receptor binding).[2] An agent's relative non-specificity may contribute to abuse. In an example from the author's practice, imipramine, with catecholamine, cholinergic and histaminergic effects, proved unsuccessful in treating a major depressive episode in a cocaine dependent patient. Contrary to instructions, the patient used the drug only intermittently for its sedative effect which precluded therapeutic levels and represented addictive behavior.

Schizophrenia

Schizophrenia with chemical dependence is argueably the most difficult to treat comorbid condition. Nearly half of individuals with schizophreniform illness have comorbid alcohol or drug problems.[3] Patients in this group more often tend to be young and male, suffer from poor living skills, and have increased likelihood of multiple substance use, violent behavior and suicide.[4]

Chronically psychotic patients may use and develop addiction to both CNS depressants and, paradoxically, psychotomimetics. With most comorbid conditions, the second disorder increases the likelihood of presentation for treatment. This is especially true of the young chronic schizophrenic group, which is twice as likely to require rehospitalization.[4] Clearly, as in all comorbid disorders, the first priority is to achieve abstinence and then initiate antipsychotic pharmacotherapy. Inpatient hospitalization is usually essential for initiating treatment and managed care approval may be more forthcoming in the dual diagnosis state than in chemical dependence alone.

Once hospitalized, if the diagnosis is at all uncertain, sparing use of antipsychotics just to manage behavior is preferable, with a taper phase to determine subsequent need. Alcoholic hallucinosis may occur in 5% of alcoholics, and stimulant or hallucinogen induced psychosis, which is not uncommon, resolves in hours to days. Therefore, prolonged antipsychotic administration may be unnecessary and side effects only serve to alienate patients from providers. Also, a watchful eye toward emergence of extrapyramidal side effects is particularly important in the young male population. Since dopamine blockers do not block cocaine or amphetamine craving or euphoria in humans, antipsychotics should be reserved for use in clear comorbid psychotic syndromes.

In most cases, standard antipsychotic doses are indicated, however, occasional interactions may warrant higher than usual doses (see Table 1 and below). Some agents may aggravate psychosis and counteract effects of antipsychotics, e.g., disulfiram, by inhibiting dopamine beta-hydroxylase, and bromocriptine and amantadine,

Table 1. Interactions Between Drugs of Abuse and Common Therapeutic Agents

Drug of abuse	Therapeutic Agent	Interaction & Mechanism (if known)
ETHANOL	•DISULFIRAM	Acetaldehyde dehydrogenase inhibition produces flushing, hypotension, nausea, tachycardia. Fatal reactions possible.
	•MAO INHIBITORS	Impaired hepatic metabolism of tyramine in some beverages produces dangerous, possibly fatal pressor response
	•TRICYCLIC ANTIDEPRESSANTS	Acute ETOH may inhibit 1st pass TCA metabolism yielding additive CNS impairment. Chronic ETOH induces hepatic TCA metabolism up to 3-fold.
	•NEUROLEPTICS	Cumulative CNS impairment on psychomotor skills, judgement & behavior. Possible increased risk of akithisia & dystonia.
	•ANTICONVULSANTS	Chronic ETOH produces prolonged hepatic microsomal enzyme induction, reducing phenytoin levels. Possible seizure risk.
BARBITURATES	•TRICYCLIC ANTIDEPRESSANTS	Increased TCA metabolism may reduce efficacy. Acutely, combination may potentiate respiratory depression.
	•MAO INHIBITORS	MAOIs may also inhibit barbiturate metabolism, prolonging intoxication.
	•NEUROLEPTICS	Induced hepatic microsomal enzymes may reduce chlorpromazine levels.
	•ANTICONVULSANTS	Valproic acid increases phenobarbital levels & toxicity. Induced hepatic microsomal enzymes may lower carbamazepine levels. Combined induction & competitive inhibition yields unpredictable phenytoin levels.
BENZODIAZEPINES	•DISULFIRAM	Inhibited hepatic oxidation may enhance BZ effects. Oxazepam & lorazepam (inactivated by glucuronidation) are not thus affected.
	•MAO INHIBITORS	2 reports of edema with chlordiazepoxide
OPIATES	•MAO INHIBITORS	Meperidine has produced severe excitation, diaphoresis, rigidity, hypertension or hypotension, coma & death.
	•NEUROLEPTICS	Chlorpromazine & meperidine may produce hypotension & excessive CNS depression.
	•ANTICONVULSANTS	Propoxyphene inhibits oxidation of carbamazepine, yielding toxic levels. Methadone metabolism may be increased by carbamazepine or phenytoin via hepatic enzyme induction, causing withdrawal.
STIMULANTS	•MAO INHIBITORS	MAOIs increase neuronal catecholamine storage; amphetamines & cocaine provoke abrupt release, hyperpyrexia, severe hypertension & death.
	•NEUROLEPTICS	Amphetamines & cocaine exacerbate positive symptoms of chronic psychosis. Conversely, neuroleptics may effectively treat stimulant-induced psychosis.

via dopamine agonism. Problems may not arise if the patient is first stabilized on an antipsychotic dose.

The combination of opiate dependence and chronic axis I disorders, especially psychosis, warrants serious consideration of methadone maintenance for initial treatment as opposed to detoxification and abstinence. Aside from the benefit of the stabilizing routine of daily outpatient methadone administration, this approach tends to be more supportive of psychotropic pharmacotherapy than abstinence oriented treatment programs.[5]

Affective Disorders

Most depressed, chemically dependent patients do not benefit from pharmacotherapy, but rather require detoxification and abstinence. Providers need to offer vigorous education and support to help patients accept that these symptoms are expectable, transient, and therefore, tolerable. In clearly diagnosed comorbid affective disorders, standard pharmacotherapy serves multiple purposes, including restoration of the euthymic state, treatment retention and relapse prevention. Standard therapeutic levels for antidepressants and lithium and adequate inhibition of platelet monoamine oxidase activity (80% reduction from baseline, for phenelzine and perhaps tranylcypromine) remain the pharmacologic objective. Important interactions between agents of abuse and treatment are listed in Table 1.

Depressed states resulting from chronic alcohol, sedative, stimulant and opiate use may meet criteria for a major syndrome transiently following the withdrawal phase. The efficacy of antidepressants in these states is not proven and antidepressant overdose is a serious risk in the event of relapse. The high rate of spontaneous remission following resolution of the withdrawal phase makes it unlikely that pharmacotherapy will be useful. Premature introduction of an agent only serves to confound the clinician's judgement about whether treatment will be needed over the longer term.

In the particular case of cocaine, recent data suggest that whether or not a discrete comorbid depression exists, post-withdrawal craving and depressive symptoms such as anhedonia may respond to some antidepressants. Such symptoms may warrant a trial, if sufficient to impair the patient's ability to participate in treatment or work. Antidepressant pharmacotherapy in these states may normalize the patient's mood, enhance treatment activity, treatment retention and early relapse prevention.[6] Conversely, desipramine has also been reported to provoke relapse in three cocaine addicts who experienced jitteriness as the agent was initiated.[7]

Some authors have reported lithium to promote cocaine abstinence in bipolar and cyclothymic patients, however this finding has not been replicated.[8,9] In any case, there is no evidence that lithium is useful for treatment in cocaine dependence without discrete comorbid bipolar disorder.

Depression is frequently reported in opiate addicts, but in most cases, antidepressants may yield no better response than placebo.[10] Longitudinal research shows that most depression in the context of methadone treatment is a transient phenomenon that may be situational or related to withdrawal.[11] Antidepressants may be useful in the fraction of methadone maintenance patients with a pre-existing or chronic major depressive disorder. Comorbid psychiatric illness in this group is associated with continued illicit drug use and increased high risk behavior for HIV transmission. Imipramine may reduce depressive symptoms in this population and may aid treatment retention and abstinence.[12]

Anxiety Disorders

In patients with chemical dependence who report anxiety symptoms, it is particularly important to determine whether these represent a discrete anxiety disorder, since anxiolytic therapy with reinforcing agents is common and poses a serious iatrogenic risk. CNS depressant withdrawal often involves a protracted phase of 3-6 months which can mimic generalized anxiety and agoraphobia. Schuckit[13] therefore maintains that even when withdrawal symptoms are sufficient to meet criteria for a major anxiety disorder, 90% of patients will spontaneously improve within weeks to the degree that pharmacotherapy will be unnecessary. Anxiety patients especially should be carefully assessed for their use of caffeine and over the counter diet pills.

Considerable data indicate that alcohol, stimulants, marijuana and hallucinogens may provoke the onset of an anxiety disorder. Many alcoholic and drug dependent patients believe they initiated substance use in an effort to self-medicate, yet there is a notable lack of objective data to support the self-medication hypothesis.[14] Also, agoraphobic patients may object to chemical dependence hospitalization, citing a fear of confinement. However, stabilization of an anxiety disorder may be extremely difficult without initial detoxification and benefit of a period of drug-free observation. A useful strategy may be to contract with the patient for intensive outpatient treatment or an extended oupatient evaluation over several weeks. If abstinence has not been achieved by the preset time, the patient will agree to reconsider voluntary hospitalization. The rapport which by this time been established with the provider, coupled with ongoing contacts from the provider during the hospitalization, may be sufficient to help the agoraphobic patient accept this disposition.

After detoxification, the first line of treatment is behavior therapy, addressing both anxiety and substance abuse with general techniques such as relaxation, meditation, and self-hypnosis and discrete techniques such as in vivo exposure for specific phobias.

Persistent, specific symptoms of panic attacks, compulsions, and the complication of major depression usually respond to appropriate conventional therapies, with the caveat that benzodiazepines are contraindicated in the dual diagnosis patient. When necessary, pharmacotherapy should therefore always begin with antidepressants. The strategy should include a contract in which the patient makes a commitment to an adequate dose for an adequate duration (usually one month), and with an understanding that side effects are usual and may require switching to one or two alternate agents before trials may be fairly concluded. Plasma levels are necessary both because of altered rates of elimination (see Table 1) and because it should not be assumed that the newly abstinent anxious patient is compliant with antidepressants when benzodiazepines may be preferred. Buspirone appears safe, may be combined with antidepressants, and is effective for generalized anxiety if the patient is vigorously educated and reminded about the slow onset and subtle perceptibility of its unique response.[15]

Benzodiazepines, despite their efficacy and safety as anxiolytics, place the anxious chemically dependent patient at risk for several reasons. These agents demonstrate cross tolerance with alcohol, barbiturates and with themselves. Single doses of benzodiazepines produce pharmacologic tolerance[16] and chronic therapeutic doses produce symptoms of physiologic dependence in up to 100% of patients.[17,18] In addition to the iatrogenic risk of substituting addictions and/or relapse by reinforcing psychological and physical dependence, treatment with these drugs in the dual diagnosis patient impedes the process of *recovery.*

Recovery from chemical dependence is distinguished from the simple state of *abstinence* as being the process of restoring intrapsychic well-being and whatever social and vocational function may have been lost as a consequence of the substance use disorder. Anxiety is normal in the recovering addict and is a therapeutic stimulus in the process of acquiring new coping behaviors. This process may require months or years of stressful effort. A comorbid anxiety disorder, however, presents excessive dysphoric challenges. Benzodiazepines, particularly those with rapid onset, e.g., alprazolam, diazepam and lorazepam, offer a degree of immediate gratification which appears to impede initiation of this effort and retention of gains. In severe conditions which prove refractory to behavioral and antidepressant approaches, a slow onset and long acting agent such as clonazepam may be the safest of this class.[19]

Personality Disorders

Personality disorders have the highest incidence of concurrent substance abuse diagnoses, especially the DSM-IIIR cluster B group (antisocial, borderline, histrionic and narcissistic), which is not surprising since antisocial and borderline personality disorders include impulsive substance use among their criteria.[20] The ECA study found some form of substance abuse/dependence in nearly 84% of individuals with antisocial personality disorder and these individuals were more likely to use drugs other than alcohol. Narcissistic, histrionic and borderline personality disorders may be found at increased prevalence rates in cocaine dependence. These patients tend to be younger, more impulsive and more prone to suicide. Their substance use may be particularly severe, yet they may benefit from inpatient chemical dependence hospitalization and Alcoholics Anonymous participation.[21]

Medication is at best only a third line treatment strategy after abstinence counseling and psychotherapy. Pharmacotherapy for these disorders has been conceptualized as a trigger reducer, based on limited support for the use of lithium, phenelzine, and fluoxetine for mood lability in cluster B disorders. In patients with these personality disorders alone, low doses of antipsychotics and carbamazepine may be useful for irritability, mood lability, anxiety, dissociative states, impulsivity, self-mutiliation, and transient psychotic symptoms. Unfortunately, virtually no careful studies have explored whether these benefits accrue to patients with comorbid chemical dependence as well. Particular caution is warranted against prolonged antipsychotic treatment (beyond 6 months) unless a drug holiday indicates clear need, because of the risk of dyskinesia.

The major problem in pharmacotherapy of comorbid chemical dependence and personality disorder may be drug seeking in the patient. Addicted patients with impaired interpersonal relations cannot help but perceive that a chemical agent offers them their most dependable relationship in life. On this basis they may suffer from intense fear of detoxification. They may cultivate sociopathic behavior as a survival skill and usually have had multiple disastrous encounters with the health care system. Many may have concurrent depressive symptoms from their addictive disorder. Finally, they may present armed with a highly developed subjective sense of drug effects and somewhat rightly perceive themselves as "amateur psychopharmacologists."

Attention Deficit Hyperactivity Disorder (ADHD)

Attention Deficit Disorder may be detected in the histories of 2 to 5% of cocaine dependent patients.[22] In its residual adult state, this disorder may require treatment because its impact on attention may cause sequelae of poor academic and job achievement. Chemically dependent adults without ADHD have not been found to benefit[23] and may develop rapid tolerance and dependence to stimulants. In cocaine addicts with ADHD, one open trial reported benefit from magnesium pemoline in terms of attentional capacity and possibly in stimulant craving.[24] Among the stimulants, magnesium pemoline is less reinforcing than others. In the addicted population, however, desipramine is recommended, since it has been effective in ADHD in children and adolescents[25] and may be useful for adults also.

Interactions of Drugs of Abuse with Psychopharmocotherapies

Drug-drug interactions are a serious concern in patients who require psychotropics for major psychiatric illnesses and who are likely to use illicit psychoactive substances concurrently with prescribed psychotropics. Table 1 presents the major medication classes used in the treatment of comorbid disorders listed according to degree of interaction with some drugs of abuse, from most to least severe.[26] These data suggest several general principles of management. Monoamine oxidase inhibitors may be contraindicated in the patient who is still at risk for using ethanol, stimulants, or meperidine. Plasma level determinations are needed at greater frequency when prescribing tricyclic antidepressants, carbamazepine or valproic acid for patients who have consumed ethanol or barbiturates heavily and/or chronically.

Other interactions may result from combinations of two therapeutic agents being used in a patient with comorbid disorders. The combination of clonidine with either chlorpromazine, haloperidol or fluphenazine has produced isolated cases of severe hypotension or delirium. Antipsychotics with bromocriptine, e.g., in a psychotic patient with severe cocaine withdrawal, would theoretically be expected to counteract each other, although this may not be a problem in a patient who is first stabilized on the antipsychotic. Trazodone added to a neuroleptic may produce hypotension.

Smoking produces numerous interactions with psychotropic agents and the incidence of nicotine dependence among chemically dependent patients probably even exceeds the high incidence among the chronic psychiatrically ill. Smoking increases the hepatic metabolism of tricyclic antidepressants; this reduction may be sufficient to reduce clinical efficacy and warrants increased scrutiny with plasma levels. Several studies report decreased phenothiazine effects in smokers, however reports of the effect of smoking on benzodiazepine dose requirements are inconclusive.[26]

Areas of Current Research

Investigations proceeding with several categories of agents may yield new approaches to the treatment of addictive diseases and comorbid disorders. One such agent is carbamazepine, with antimanic and anti-kindling effects that may provide unique benefits for patients with recurrent cyclothymia/mania, prolonged cocaine craving and cocaine-induced paranoia.[27]

Anti-appetitive use is a potential but largely untested application of pharmacotherapy in chemical dependence which includes reducing craving and other drug seeking traits. This role is suggested by experiments in which animals have been trained to self-administer a drug of abuse and subsequently decrease or cease self-administration after the introduction of a therapeutic agent. Such agents may also have concurrent efficacy for other psychiatric syndromes, which would make them parsimonious choices for patients with some dual disorders. For example, the serotonin uptake inhibitors, which are effective antidepressants, have also been proposed to posess anti-appetitive effects for alcohol.[28] The mixed opiate agonist-antagonist buprenorphine appears to reduce both heroin and cocaine use in humans with combined heroin and cocaine dependence[29] and is under preliminary investigation for use in treating refractory depression.[30] Mechanisms for anti-appetitive effects still remain largely unknown.

Management Principles

Finally, the complexity of these disorders warrants exceptional care in assessment, which depends on the temporal relationships between symptoms and alcohol and drug use and longitudinal evaluation of treatment response. Dual diagnosis is an important factor in relapse in chemical dependence, yet there is some evidence that treatment matching based on psychiatric severity improves outcome.[5,31] Inpatient treatment is recommended for both its medical and cost effectiveness as the best way to obtain immediate, complete abstinence, compliance, treatment response data, and long term recovery skills.[32,33] If available, a medically-managed facility with specific programming for dual diagnoses is optimal, and should permit an adequate length of stay to permit resolution of withdrawal and initial pharmacotherapy response.[33] Managed care reviews may approve dual diagnosis patients for initial inpatient admission if the following criteria are clearly documented: (1) moderate to severe dependence, (2) dysfunction and likely losses, (3) medical or psychiatric risk such as potential suicide gesture, and (4) rehabilitation potential.

A psychoeducational treatment model is especially valuable to dual diagnosis patients and their families because of their own confusion about symptom causality, therapeutic vs. abused drugs, and prognosis. This approach lends structure to the initial treatment, destigmatizes the two illnesses, and helps patients and families reduce the additional risk factors of guilt and blame. The management of pharmacotherapy in these disorders involves active, directive education on the part of the psychiatrist, taking the definitive stance of helping the patient to protect him/herself from his/her disease.

The clinician does not expect a smooth course, and tells the patient so, forewarning that when relapse occurs, rational practice is to intensify treatment, e.g., increasing self help activity, adding drug counseling or group therapy to individual pharmacotherapy, or inpatient rehabilitation. Table 2 outlines vital components of a pharmacotherapy contract for dual diagnosis patients. Underlying these issues is the essential need for continual reevaluation of the patient's condition in terms of medication response and active treatment participation. The latter involves initiating lifestyle changes such as participating in a self-help group, utilizing sober supports such as a

---

Table 2:

Key components of a pharmacotherapy contract in the dual diagnosis patient

1. Medication is part of a rational psychosocial treatment "package", and will be discontinued if key psychosocial components are neglected.

2. Urine or blood testing may be required at any time to provide an independent source of data about the course of the chemical dependence, or to determine if prescribed medication is reaching adequate levels in blood.

3. Medication will be used only as prescribed. Any need for changes will first be discussed with the physician. A unilateral change in medication by the patient often is an early sign of relapse.

4. Changes in medication will be prescribed one at a time, e.g. two agents will not be initiated simultaneously.

5. When used, the purpose of medication is to treat predetermined target symptoms. If medication proves ineffective for these, it will be discontinued.

6. Once target symptoms remit, a process of dose tapering may be initiated to determine the minimum dose necessary to maintain healthy function. Periodically, the medication strategy will include a period of discontinuation, or "drug holiday". Medication may not be necessary on a long term basis.

sponsor(s), and engaging in longitudinal (i.e., aftercare) treatment for both addiction and the comorbid illness. Patients with comorbid addiction and other psychiatric disorders who participate in these modalities often have gratifying responses to pharmacotherapy when indicated.

REFERENCES

1. Kosten TR, Kleber HD. Differential diagnosis of psychiatric comorbidity in substance abusers. J Subst Abuse Treat. 1988; 5:201-6.

2. Ciraulo DA, Shader RI. *Clinical Manual of Chemical Dependence.* Washington DC: American Psychiatric Press, 1991.

3. Regier DA, Farmer ME, Rae DS, Locke BZ, Keith SJ, Judd LL, Goodwin FK. Comorbidity of mental disorders with alcohol and other drug abuse. Arch Gen Psychiatry. 1990; 264:2511-8.

4. Caton C, Gralnick A, Bender S, Simon R. Young chronic patients and substance abuse. Hosp Comm Psychiat. 1989; 40:1037- 40.

5. McLellan AT, Luborsky L, Woody GE, OBrien CP, Druley KA. Predicting response to alcohol and drug abuse treatments. Arch Gen Psychiatry. 1983; 40:620-625.

6. Gawin FH, Kleber HD, Byck R, Rounsaville BJ, Kosten TR, Jatlow PI, Morgan C. Desipramine facilitation of initial cocaine abstinence. Arch Gen Psychiatry. 1989; 46:117-21.

7. Weiss R. Relapse to cocaine abuse after initiating desipramine treatment. JAMA. 1988; 260:2545-6.

8. Nunes E, McGrath P, Wager S, Quitkin FM. Lithium treatment for cocaine abusers with bipolar spectrum disorders. Am J Psychiatry. 1990; 147:655-7.

9. Lemere F. Lithium treatment of cocaine addiction. Am J Psychiatry. 1991; 148:276.

10. Kleber HD, Weissman MM, Rounsaville BJ. Imipramine as treatment for depression in addicts. Arch Gen Psychiatry. 1983; 40:649-53.

11. Rounsaville BJ, Kosten TR, Kleber HD. Long-term changes in current psychiatric diagnoses of treated opiate addicts. Compr Psychiatry. 1986; 27:480-98.

12. Nunes EV, Quitkin FM, Brady R, Stewart JW. Imipramine treatment of methadone maintenance patients with affective disorder and illicit drug use. Am J Psychiatry. 1991; 148:667-9.

13. Schuckit M, Irwin M, Brown S. The history of anxiety symptoms among 171 primary alcoholics. J Stud Alcohol. 1990; 51:34-41.

14. Cox BJ, Norton GR, Dorward J, Fergusson PA. The relationship between panic attacks and chemical dependencies. Addict Behav. 1989; 14:53-60.

15. Gastfriend DR, Rosenbaum JR. Adjunctive buspirone in benzodiazepine treatment of four patients with panic disorder. Am J Psychiatry. 1989; 146:914-6.

16. Greenblatt DJ, Shader RI. Dependence, tolerance, and addiction to benzo-diazepines: clinical and pharmacokinetic considerations. Drug Metab Rev. 1978; 8:13-28.

17. Busto U, Sellers EM, Naranjo CA, Cappell, H, Sanchez, Craig M, Sykora, K. Withdrawal reaction after long-term therapeutic use of benxodiazepines. NEJM. 1986; 315:854-9.

18. Rickels K, Schweizer E, Case WG, Greenblatt DJ. Long-term therapeutic use of benzodiazepines. I. Effects of abrupt discontinuation. Arch Gen Psychiatry. 1990; 47:99-907.

19. Herman JB, Rosenbaum JF, Brotman AW. The alprazolam to clonazepam switch for the treatment of panic disorder. J Clin Psychopharmacol. 1987; 7:175-8.

20. Akiskal H, Chen S, Davis G, Puzantian V, Kashgarian M, Bolinger J. Bor-derline: an adjective in search of a noun. J Clin Psychiatry. 1985; 46:41-8.

21. Nace E, Davis C, Gaspari J. Axis II comorbidity in substance abuse. Am J Psychiatry. 1991; 148:118-20.

22. Weiss RD, Mirin SM, Michael JL, Sollogub AC. Psychopathology in chronic cocaine abusers. Am J Drug Alcohol Abuse. 1986; 12:17- 29.

23. Gawin FH, Riordan, Kleber HD. Methylphenidate treatment of cocaine abusers without attention deficit disorder: a negative report. Am J Drug Alc Abuse. 1985; 11:193-7.

24. Weiss RD, Pope HD, Mirin SM. Treatment of chronic cocaine abuse and attention deficit disorder, residual type, with magnesium pemoline. Drug Alc Dep. 1985; 15:69-72.

25. Gastfriend DR, Biederman J, Jellinek M. Desipramine in the treatment of adolescents with attention deficit disorder. Am J Psychiatry. 1984; 141:906-8.

26. Hansten PD, Horn JR. *Drug Interactions and Updates: A clinical perspec-tive and analysis of current developments.* Malvern PA: Lea & Fibiger, 1990.

27. Halikas JA, Crosby RD, Carlson GA, Crea F, Graves NM, Bowers LD. Co-caine reduction in unmotivated crack users using carbamazepine versus placebo in a short-term, double-blind crossover design. Clin Pharmacol Ther. 1991; 50:81-95.

28. Naranjo CA, Sellers EM, Sullivan JT, Woodley DV, Kadlec K, Sykora K. The serotonin uptake inhibitor citalopram attenuates ethanol intake. Clin Pharm Ther. 1987; 41:266-74.

29. Gastfriend DR, Mendelson JH, Mello NK, Teoh SK. Preliminary results of an open trial of buprenorphine in the outpatient treatment of combined heroin and cocaine dependence. NIDA Research Monograph Series: Problems of Drug De-pendence 1991, in press.

30. Bodkin JA, Zornberg GL, Lukas S, Cole JO. Buprenorphine treatment of refractory depression. J Clin Psychopharm, in press.

31. Miller W, Hester R. Matching problem drinkers with optimal treatments. In Miller W, Hester R (Ed.), *Treating Addictive Behaviors: Processes of Change.* New York: Plenum Press, 1986.

32. Chapman-Walsh D, Hingson RW, Merrigan DM, Levenson S, Cupples A, Heeren T, Coffman GA, Becker CA, Barker TA, Hamilton SK, McGuire TG, Kelly CA. A randomized trial of treatment options for alcohol-abusing workers. NEJM. 1991; 325:775-82.

33. Hoffman NG, Halikas JA, Mee-Lee D, Weedman RD. *Patient Placement Criteria for the Treatment of Psychoactive Substance Use Disorders*. Washington D.C.: American Society of Addiction Medicine, 1991.

SELECTIVE GUIDE TO CURRENT REFERENCE SOURCES ON TOPICS DISCUSSED IN THIS ISSUE

Comorbidity of Addictive and Psychiatric Disorders

Lynn Kasner Morgan, MLS
James E. Raper, Jr., MSLS

Each issue of *Journal of Addictive Diseases* features a section offering suggestions on where to look for further information on included topics. In this issue, our intent is to guide readers to selec-

Lynn Kasner Morgan is Assistant Professor of Medical Education, Assistant Dean for Information Resources and Systems, and Director of the Gustave L. and Janet W. Levy Library of the Mount Sinai Medical Center, Inc. James E. Raper, Jr., is Instructor in Medical Education and Assistant Director for Technical Services at Mount Sinai, One Gustave L. Levy Place, New York, NY 10029-6574.

[Haworth co-indexing entry note]: Selective Guide to Current Reference Sources: "Comorbidity of Addictive and Psychiatric Disorders." Morgan, Lynn Kasner, and James E. Raper, Jr.. Co-published simultaneously in *Journal of Addictive Diseases,* (The Haworth Press, Inc.) Vol. 12, No. 3, 1993, pp. 171-185; and: *Comorbidity of Addictive and Psychiatric Disorders* (Ed: Norman S. Miller, and Barry Stimmel) The Haworth Press, Inc., 1993, pp. 171-185. Multiple copies of this article/chapter may be purchased from The Haworth Document Delivery Center. Call 1-800-3-HAWORTH (1-800-342-9678) between 9:00 - 5:00(EST) and ask for DOCUMENT DELIVERY CENTER.

tive substantive sources of current information on comorbidity of addictive and psychiatric disorders.

Some published reference works utilize designated terminology (controlled vocabularies) which must be used to find material on topics of interest. For these a sample of available search terms has been indicated to assist the reader in accessing suitable sources for his/her purposes. Other reference tools use keywords or free-text terms from the title of the document, the abstract, and the name of any responsible agency or conference. In searching using keywords, be sure to look under all possible synonyms to retrieve the concept in question.

An asterisk (*) appearing before a published source indicates that all or part of that source is in machine-readable form and can be accessed through an online database search. Database searching is recommended for retrieving sources of information that coordinate multiple variables, concepts, or subject areas. Most health sciences libraries offer database services which can include mediated online searching, access to locally mounted datafiles, front-end software packages, and CD-ROM technology. Searching can also be done from one's office or home with subscriptions to database services and microcomputers equipped with modems.

In addition to bibliographic sources, there are also local, state, and national agencies that provide alcohol and drug information and referral services. A major agency within the United States Government is OSAP's National Clearinghouse for Alcohol and Drug Information (ONCADI), P.O. Box 2345, Rockville, MD 20847-2345; 1-800-729-6686; TDD 1-800-487-4889; extended operating hours–9 a.m. to 7 p.m. Eastern time, Monday through Friday; FAX 301-468-6433.

ONCADI was established by the Office of Substance Abuse Prevention (OSAP) as the central point within the Federal Government for current print and audiovisual materials about alcohol and other drugs. ONCADI answers more than 18,000 telephone and mail inquiries each month and distributes some 18 million printed items a year.

ONCADI's resources include scientific findings; databases on prevention programs and materials, field experts, and federal grants information; materials tailored to parents, teachers, youth, and others; and information about organizations and groups concerned with alcohol and other drug problems. ONCADI shares these resources with the public, including healthcare practitioners and researchers, through the following services:

1. Response to telephone, mail, and in-person information requests
2. Comprehensive alcohol and other drug resource referrals
3. Free, customized database searches
4. Availability of on-site library research
5. *Prevention Pipeline*, a bimonthly publication filled with the latest information about prevention research, resources, and activities in the field
6. Grant announcements and application kits

ONCADI also supports OSAP's Regional Alcohol and Drug Awareness Resource Network (RADAR), which is comprised of State clearinghouses and specialized information centers of national organizations.

Readers are encouraged to consult their librarians for further assistance before undertaking research on a topic.

Suggestions regarding the content and organization of this section are welcome and should be sent to the authors.

1. INDEXING AND ABSTRACTING SOURCES

Place of publication, publisher, start date, frequency of publication, and brief descriptions are noted.

Biological Abstracts (1926-) and *Biological Abstracts/RRM* (v.18, 1980-). Philadelphia, BioSciences Information Service, semi-monthly. Reports on worldwide research in the life sciences.

> See: Concept headings for abstracts, such as behavioral biology, pharmacology, psychiatry, public health, and toxicology sections.

> See: Keyword-in-context subject index.

Chemical Abstracts. Columbus, Ohio, American Chemical Society, 1907- , weekly. A key to the world's literature of chemistry and chemical engineering, including serial publications, proceedings and edited collections, technical reports, dissertations, new book and audiovisual materials announcements, and patent documents.

See: *Index Guide* for cross-referencing and indexing policies.

See: *General Subject Index* terms, such as drug dependence; drug interactions; drug tolerance; epidemiology; ethanol, biologic studies; mental activity, mental disorder; psychotropics.

See: Keyword subject indexes.

Criminal Justice Periodical Index. Ann Arbor, Mich., Indexing Services, University Microfilms, 1975- , 3 times per year, including annual cumulation. Covers more than 100 English-language journals in criminology, including alcoholism and drug abuse.

See: Keyword subject index.

Dissertation Abstracts International. Section B. The Sciences and Engineering. Ann Arbor, Mich., University Microfilms, v.30, 1969/70- , monthly. Includes author-prepared abstracts of doctoral dissertations from 500 participating institutions throughout North America and the world. A separate section contains European dissertations.

See: Keyword subject index.

Excerpta Medica. Amsterdam, The Netherlands, Excerpta Medica Foundation, 1947- , 45 subject sections. A major abstracting service covering more than 4,300 biomedical journals. The abstracts, including English summaries for non-English-language articles, appear in one or more of the published subject sections, excluding Section 37, *Drug Literature Index,* and Section 38, *Adverse Reactions Titles,* which are indexes only. Each of the sections has a comprehensive subject index. Since 1978 all the *Excerpta Med-*

ica sections have been available for computer searching in the integrated online file, EMBASE.

Particularly relevant to the topics in this issue are Section 40, *Drug Dependence, Alcohol Abuse and Alcoholism;* Section 22, *Human Genetics;* and the sections that have addiction, alcoholism, or drug subdivisions: Section 130, *Clinical Pharmacology;* Section 30, *Pharmacology;* Section 32, *Psychiatry;* and Section 17, *Public Health, Social Medicine and Epidemiology.*

*Index Medicus (includes *Bibliography of Medical Reviews*). Bethesda, Md., National Library of Medicine, 1960- , monthly, with annual cumulations. Published as author and subject indexes to more than 3,000 journals in the biomedical sciences. Subject headings are based on the controlled vocabulary or thesaurus, *Medical Subject Headings* (MeSH). Since 1966 it has been produced from the MEDLARS database, which provides more comprehensive retrieval, including keyword access and English-language abstracts, than its printed counterparts: *Index Medicus, International Nursing Index,* and *Index to Dental Literature.*

> See: *MeSH* terms, such as affective disorders; alcohol, ethyl; alcoholism; anxiety disorders; comorbidity; compulsive behavior; depressive disorder; drug therapy; drug utilization; eating disorders; epidemiology; family; gambling; genetics; inpatients; mental disorders; obsessive-compulsive disorders; outpatients; psychiatry; psychotropic drugs; risk factors; substance abuse; substance dependence; substance use disorders; treatment outcome.

Index to Scientific Reviews. Philadelphia, Institute for Scientific Information, 1974- , semiannual.

> See: Permuterm keyword subject index.

> See: Citation index.

*International Pharmaceutical Abstracts. Washington, D.C., American Society of Hospital Pharmacists, 1964- , semimonthly. A key to the world's literature of pharmacy.

See: IPA subject terms, such as alcoholism, controlled substance analogs, dependence, drug abuse, drug withdrawal, epidemiology; psychotic disorders.

Psychological Abstracts. Washington, D.C., American Psychological Association, 1927- , monthly. A compilation of nonevaluative summaries of the world's literature in psychology and related disciplines.

See: Index terms, such as addiction, alcohol abuse, alcohol psychosis, alcoholism, anxiety neurosis, comorbidity, drug abuse, drug addiction, drug dependency, drug interactions, drug usage, drug usage screening, epidemiology, mental disorders, pathological gambling psychosis.

Public Affairs Information Service Bulletin. New York, Public Affairs Information Service, v.55, 1969- , semimonthly. An index to informational resources in the field of public affairs and public policy published throughout the world.

See: *PAIS* subject headings, such as alcoholism, drug abuse, drug addicts, drugs, mental health, mental illness, narcotics, psychotropic drugs.

Science Citation Index. Philadelphia, Institute for Scientific Information, 1961- , bimonthly.

See: Permuterm keyword subject index.

See: Citation index.

Social Planning/Policy & Development Abstracts. San Diego, Calif., Sociological Abstracts, Inc., v.6, 1984- , semiannual.

See: Thesaurus and descriptors listed under *Sociological Abstracts.*

Social Work Research and Abstracts. New York, National Association of Social Workers, v.13, 1977- , quarterly. Combines original research reports in the field of social welfare with abstracts of articles previously published in social work and related fields.

See: Fields of service sections, such as health and health care, substance use and abuse/alcoholism.

See: Subject index.

Sociological Abstracts. San Diego, Calif ., Sociological Abstracts, Inc., 1952- , 6 times per year. A collection of nonevaluative abstracts which reflect the world's serial literature in sociology and related disciplines.

See: *Thesaurus of Sociological Indexing Terms.*

See: Descriptors such as alcohol use, alcoholism, behavior problems, drug abuse, drug addiction, drug use, epidemiology, mental health, mental illness, psychosis, substance abuse.

Substance Abuse Index and Abstracts: A Guide to Drug. Alcohol and Tobacco Research:, New York, Scientific DataLink, 1989-, annual with supplements. A multidisciplinary guide to the literature on psychoactive substance use and abuse, prevention, treatment, and control.

See: Subject index.

2. CURRENT AWARENESS PUBLICATIONS

Current Contents: Clinical Medicine. Philadelphia, Institute for Scientific Information, v.15, 1987- , weekly.

See: Keyword index.

Current Contents: Life Sciences. Philadelphia, Institute for Scientific Information, v.10, 1967- , weekly.

See: Keyword index.

Current Contents: Social & Behavioral Sciences. Philadelphia, Institute for Scientific Information, v.6, 1974- , weekly.

> See: Keyword index.

3. BOOKS

Andrews, Theodora. *A Bibliography of Drug Abuse, Including Alcohol and Tobacco.* Littleton, Colo., Libraries Unlimited, 1977-

Andrews, Theodora. *Guide to the Literature of Pharmacy and the Pharmaceutical Sciences.* Littleton, Colo., Libraries Unlimited, 1986.

Bibliography of Abstracts on Coexisting Substance Abuse and Mental Disorders. Rockville, Md., U.S. Alcohol, Drug Abuse, and Mental Health Administration, Office for Treatment Improvement, 1990.

Cocaine: An Annotated Bibliography. Jackson, Research Institute of Pharmaceutical Sciences, University of Mississippi and University Press of Mississippi, c1988.

Lowinson, Joyce H., ed. [and others]. *Substance Abuse: A Comprehensive Textbook.* 2nd ed. Baltimore, Williams & Wilkins, c1992.

Medical and Health Care Books and Serials in Print: An Index to Literature in the Health Sciences. New York, R. R. Bowker Co., annual.

> See: Library of Congress subject headings, such as alcohol, alcoholism, drug abuse, drugs, narcotic habit, psychotropic drugs.

Miller, Norman S., ed. *Comprehensive Handbook of Drug and Alcohol Addiction.* New York, Dekker, c1991.

National Library of Medicine Current Catalog. Bethesda, Md., National Library of Medicine, 1966- , quarterly, with annual cumulations.

See: *MeSH* terms as noted in Section 1 under *Index Medicus.*

O'Brien, Robert [and others]. *The Encyclopedia of Drug Abuse.* 2nd ed. New York, Facts on File, c1992.

O'Brien, Robert and Morris Chafetz. *The Encyclopedia of Alcoholism.* 2nd ed. New York, Facts on File, c1991.

Page, Penny B. *Alcohol Use and Alcoholism: A Guide to the Literature.* New York, Garland Publishing, 1986.

Stimmel, Barry [and others]. *The Facts About Drug Use: Coping with Drug Use in Your Family, at Work, in Your Community.* Mount Vernon, N.Y., Consumers's Union, c1991.

World Health Organization Catalogue: New Books. Geneva, World Health Organization, annual (supplements World Health Organization Publications and includes periodicals).

4. U.S. GOVERNMENT PUBLICATIONS

*Monthly Catalog of United States Government Publications. Washington, D.C., U.S. Government Printing Office, 1895- , monthly.

See: Following agencies: Alcohol, Drug Abuse and Mental Health Administration; Centers for Disease Control; Food and Drug Administration; National Cancer Institute; National Center for Health Statistics; National Institute of Mental Health; National Institute on Drug Abuse; National Institutes of Health.

See: Subject headings, derived chiefly from the Library of Congress, such as alcohol, alcoholics, alcoholism, drug abuse, drug habit, drug interactions, drug utilization, drug dependence, drugs, epidemiology, medical genetics, narcotics, pharmacology, psychiatry.

See: Title index.

5. ONLINE BIBLIOGRAPHIC DATABASES

Only those databases which have no print counterparts are included in this section. Print sources which have online database equivalents are noted throughout this guide by the asterisk (*) which appears before the title. If you do not have direct access to these databases, consult your librarian for assistance.

ALCOHOL AND ALCOHOL PROBLEMS SCIENCE DATABASE: ETOH (National Institute on Alcohol Abuse and Alcoholism, Rockville, Md.).

Use: Keywords.

ALCOHOL INFORMATION FOR CLINICIANS AND EDUCATORS (Project Cork Institute, Dartmouth Medical School, Hanover, N.H.)

Use: Keywords.

ASI: AMERICAN STATISTICS INDEX (Congressional Information Services, Inc., Washington, D.C.).

Use: Keywords.

DRUG INFORMATION FULLTEXT (American Society of Hospital Pharmacists, Bethesda, Md.).

Use: Keywords.

DRUGINFO AND ALCOHOL USE AND ABUSE (Hazelden Foundation, Center City, Minn., and Drug Information Service Center, College of Pharmacy, University of Minnesota, Minneapolis, Minn.).

Use: Keywords.

FAMILY RESOURCES DATABASE (National Council on Family Relations and Inventory of Marriage and Family Literature Project, Minneapolis, Minn.).

Use: Keywords.

LEXIS (Mead Data Central, Inc., Dayton, Ohio).

Use: Keywords.

MAGAZINE INDEX (Information Access Co., Belmont, Calif.).

Use: Keywords.

MEDICAL AND PSYCHOLOGICAL PREVIEWS: MPPS (BRS Bibliographic Retrieval Services, Inc., McLean, Va.).

Use: Keywords.

MENTAL HEALTH ABSTRACTS (IFI/Plenum Data Co., Alexandria, Va.).

Use: Keywords.

NATIONAL NEWSPAPER INDEX (Information Access Co., Belmont, Calif.).

Use: Keywords.

NTIS (National Technical Information Service, U.S. Dept. of Commerce, Springfield, Va.).

Use: Keywords.

PSYCINFO (American Psychological Association, Washington, D.C.).

Use: Keywords.

WESTLAW (West Publishing Co., St. Paul, Minn.)

Use: Keywords.

6. HANDBOOKS, DIRECTORIES, GRANT SOURCES, ETC.

Annual Register of Grant Support. Wilmette, Ill., National Register Pub. Co., annual.

> See: Internal medicine, medicine; pharmacology; psychiatry, psychology, mental health sections.

> See: Subject index.

Biomedical Index to PHS-Supported Research. Bethesda, Md., National Institutes of Health, Division of Research Grants, annual.

> See: Subject index.

Database Directory. White Plains, N.Y., Knowledge Industry Publications in cooperation with the American Society for Information Science, annual.

> See: Subject index.

Directory of Online Databases (includes *Online Databases in the Medical and Life Sciences*). New York, Cuadra/Elsevier, quarterly

> See: Subject index.

Directory of Research Grants. Phoenix, Ariz., Oryx Press, annual.

> See: Subject index terms, such as alcoholism, drug abuse.

Encyclopedia of Associations. Detroit, Gale Research, annual (occasional supplements between editions).

> See: Subject index.

Foundation Directory. New York, The Foundation Center, biennial (updated between editions by *Foundation Directory Supplement*).

> See: Index of foundations.

> See: Index of foundations by state and city.

> See: Index of donors, trustees, and administrators.

See: Index of fields of interest.

Health Hotlines: Toll-Free Numbers from DIRLINE. Bethesda, Md., National Library of Medicine, 1990.

Information Industry Directory. Detroit, Gale Research, annual.

National Guide to Funding in Health. 2nd ed. New York, The Foundation Center, 1990.

National Treatment Resource Issue of Alcoholism & Addiction Treatment Programs, Including Agencies, Services, & Community Resources. 8th ed. (*Addiction & Recovery*, v.12, no.5). Cleveland, Ohio, International Publishing Group, 1991.

Roper, Fred W. and Jo Anne Boorkman. Introduction to *Reference Sources in the Health Sciences.* 2nd ed. Chicago, Medical Library Association, c1984.

The SALIS Directory: Substance Abuse Librarians and Information Specialists. 2nd ed. Berkeley, Calif ., Alcohol Research Group, Medical Research Institute of San Francisco and University of California, Berkeley, 1991.

Statistics Sources. Detroit, Gale Research, annual.

7. JOURNAL LISTINGS

Ulrich's International Periodicals Directory, Now Including Irregular Serials & Annuals. New York, R. R. Bowker Co., annual (supplemented between editions by Ulrich's Update).

See: Subject categories, such as drug abuse and alcoholism, medical sciences, pharmacy and pharmacology, psychology.

8. AUDIOVISUAL PROGRAMS

The Directory of Medical Video Programs. Hawthorne, N.J., Ridge Publishing Co., 1990.

National Library of Medicine Audiovisuals Catalog. Bethesda, Md., National Library of Medicine, 1977- , quarterly, with annual cumulations.

See: *MeSH* terms as noted in Section 1 under *Index Medicus.*

Patient Education Sourcebook. 2 v. Saint Louis, Mo., Health Sciences Communications Association, c1985-90.

See: *MeSH* terms as noted in Section 1 under *Index Medicus.*

9. GUIDES TO UPCOMING MEETINGS

Scientific Meetings. San Diego, Calif., Scientific Meetings Publications, quarterly.

See: Subject indexes.

See: Association listing.

World Meetings: Medicine. New York, Macmillan Pub. Co., quarterly.

See: Keyword index.

See: Sponsor directory and index.

World Meetings: Outside United States and Canada. New York, Macmillan Pub. Co., quarterly.

See: Keyword index.

See: Sponsor directory and index.

World Meetings: United States and Canada. New York, Macmillan Pub. Co., quarterly.

See: Keyword index.

See: Sponsor directory and index.

10. PROCEEDINGS OF MEETINGS

Conference Pacers Index. Louisville, Ky., Data Courier, v.6, 1978- , monthly.

Directory of Published Proceedings. Series SEMT. Science/Engineering/Medicine/Technology. White Plains, N.Y., InterDok Corp., v.3, 1967- , monthly, except July-August, with annual cumulations.

Index to Scientific and Technical Proceedings. Philadelphia, Institute for Scientific Information, 1978- , monthly with semiannual cumulations.

11. SPECIALIZED RESEARCH CENTERS

Medical Research Centres. Harlow, Essex, Longman, biennial.

International Research Centers Directory. Detroit, Gale Research, annual.

Research Centers Directory. Detroit, Gale Research, annual (updated by *New Research Centers*).

12. SPECIAL LIBRARY COLLECTIONS

Directory of Special Libraries and Information Centers. Detroit, Gale Research, annual (updated by *New Special Libraries*).